The Cleveland Clinic Guide to

HEART
ATTACKS

Also in the *Cleveland Clinic Guide* Series

The Cleveland Clinic Guide to

HEART ATTACKS

Curtis Mark Rimmerman, MD, MBA, FACC

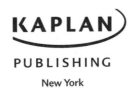

KAPLAN

PUBLISHING

New York

Artwork is reprinted with the permission of The Cleveland Clinic Center for Medical Art & Photograph © 2009.

Published by Kaplan Publishing, a division of Kaplan, Inc.
1 Liberty Plaza, 24th Floor
New York, NY 10006

Printed in the United States of America

10 9 8 7 6 5 4 3 2 1

The Library of Congress Cataloging-in-Publication Data has been applied for.

ISBN-13: 978-1-4277-9968-5

Kaplan Publishing books are available at special quantity discounts to use for sales promotions, employee premiums, or educational purposes. Please email our Special Sales Department to order or for more information at *kaplanpublishing@kaplan.com,* or write to Kaplan Publishing, 1 Liberty Plaza, 24th Floor, New York, NY 10006.

Contents

Introduction

J ust below this short paragraph, sitting alone in a sea of white, is a dot. If I've caught your attention, you're likely wondering why a cardiologist is focusing his attention on a dot. Maybe you're thinking it represents a blood cell or possibly a microchip for some fancy heart device. However, it's way too big to be a blood cell; as for the latter, I have no idea how big or small microchips are.

•

The dot is just a few millimeters in diameter, just a fraction of an inch. If I told you that the dot could kill, you might be slightly more interested in reading on. But before explaining the story behind the dot, I want to transport you for a minute to one of my exam rooms. There you are, sitting on the exam table, wearing one of those unflattering hospital gowns and wishing you were any place other than in an exam room. I tell you that you have coronary artery disease and that you are at risk for a heart attack. I go on to say that you really need to start making some changes in your life and that you're going to have to alter your diet, quit smoking, take up exercise, and possibly even begin taking cholesterol-lowering drugs. Instead of droning on, I can pretty much guarantee that you'd be far more interested in hearing my explanation of the dot than hearing any tedious admonishments about "lifestyle" changes.

So here's the story on the dot. The dot is similar in size to the clots that develop when a small mound of plaque in a coronary artery cracks open. When this happens, the body responds by trying to repair the fissure and, in doing so, simply makes the mound bigger. In fact, often the repair grows large enough to snuff off blood flow, so that the portion of heart tissue downstream from the clot, which is served by that artery, will quickly begin to starve. The flow of red blood cells, which are packed with oxygen, has been reduced to a trickle, and the heart muscle cells that rely on a constant supply of blood begin to die.

This is a heart attack—initially caused by clots the size of that tiny dot.

Unfortunately, for too many people, a heart attack is often the first sign of the existence of coronary artery disease. Many times, it is also a lethal first sign. Although the risk of developing coronary artery disease can be determined at birth—meaning that through no fault of your own, you've inherited genes that predispose you to the development of heart disease—you have far more control over the matter than you might imagine.

This book is written for anyone interested in heart disease and heart attack, regardless of health status or age. You will learn about all aspects of heart disease: how it develops (and how to minimize the likelihood of that happening); how it can affect heart structures; and how it is managed using nonmedical, medical, surgical, and interventional strategies.

This book also is meant to get your attention about that dot, because, as I've said, there are fundamental steps you can take to help minimize your chances of heart attack. Will they involve sacrifice? Of course. But you don't have to swear off every food you love, and you don't have to train like an Olympian. Much of it is common sense and discipline. Thankfully, discipline has a way of quickly making routines second nature. Most of us don't think twice anymore about putting on a seat belt when we get into a car; if we have children, you better believe we'll strap them in.

Inconvenient? Hardly. Worth the effort? Completely. This is how you should approach lifestyle changes—somewhat inconvenient at the outset but worth their weight in gold in terms of what they offer in health and longevity.

Think of your health as a healthcare retirement account. You wouldn't spend all of your retirement savings in one day. By apportioning your lifestyle improvements over your lifetime, you will significantly improve your chances of realizing a longer and happier life free of chronic disease including heart disease. Diet and exercise are commonly recommended and make complete sense. Finding the motivation and maintaining the discipline to sustain these efforts over a period of years is more difficult. It is my hope that educating yourself about heart disease and learning how to preempt the manifestations of heart disease such as heart attack will provide you impetus for sustained change. That, in a nutshell, is the purpose of this book.

Curtis Mark Rimmerman, MD, MBA, FACC
Gus P. Karos Chair in Clinical Cardiovascular Medicine
Staff Cardiologist
Department of Cardiovascular Medicine
Heart and Vascular Institute
Cleveland Clinic
Cleveland, Ohio USA

Chapter 1

What Is Heart Disease?

L ike a lion stalking its prey, coronary artery disease can sneak up on you in a silent, deadly manner.

It progresses silently into the heart's arteries, and when symptoms develop—like significant chest pain or sensations of indigestion—they aren't always recognized as warning signals for heart disease or heart problems.

• • • *Fast Fact* • • •

Heart disease begins in early childhood. Autopsies on young accident victims have identified "fatty streaks," cholesterol deposits within the aorta, as early as the teenage years.

• • •

For some people, the first sign of heart disease is a heart attack, and it can be a lethal one. A person can feel great one day and suddenly die the next. When this happens to someone we know, it reminds us that heart disease and lethal heart attacks can strike anyone, regardless of age, gender, or fitness status.

Additional Info

It's important to have your fasting cholesterol and blood fats checked and also to have a fasting blood sugar test. It is recommended that this start at age 25 years—earlier if there is a prominent family history of heart disease, vascular disease, or diabetes.

Unfortunately, too many people believe that a heart attack is unpredictable and inevitable. *It's not as if I can do anything about it. So why bother worrying or changing my lifestyle?*

Doctors find this fatalistic attitude troubling. For sure, we can't predict who'll have a heart attack, but we can easily identify patients who are more likely to be candidates. We can then educate them about lifestyle changes that will significantly cut their risks of heart attack: quitting smoking, eating healthier, and exercising regularly.

• • • *Fast Fact* • • •

Individuals who suffer a heart attack are much more likely to experience a second heart attack compared to the general population. Second heart attacks are typically more life threatening as the heart is already damaged and less normal heart muscle is available to sustain the heart's output of blood.

• • •

Yet even when such advice is given, it often goes unheeded. People change their behavior, but old habits are difficult to place aside. Even more disturbing, patients at the highest risk often don't see a physician or get medical care until they actually experience a heart attack. Survivors are lucky, because heart attacks can—and do—kill. It's doubly important that survivors of a heart attack intensify their lifestyle modification efforts.

Despite a greater understanding of heart disease and vigorous efforts to educate the public, myths about heart disease and heart attack stay with us.

Common Misconceptions About Heart Disease

If I Don't Have Symptoms, Might I Still Have Heart Disease?

Since many diseases have early warning signs or symptoms, it's understandable that people believe this is the case with heart disease. But it's absolutely untrue. In fact, many people with significant obstructive coronary artery disease—that is, plaque buildup on the insides of heart artery walls, which reduces blood flow—have no symptoms at all until their first heart attack. Even critical blockages can render no symptoms in up to 30 to 40 percent of cases. This is termed silent myocardial ischemia, also known as deficient oxygen delivery to the heart muscle, creating an imbalance between oxygen supply and demand. So believing that an absence of symptoms means that we are safe from heart disease or heart attack is wrong, wrong, wrong.

If My Parents Had Heart Disease, Am I Doomed?

Even if your parents had or have heart disease, you may not develop heart disease. Genetics certainly plays a role, but it's the combination of genes you inherit that dictates what happens down the road. You are a unique combination of your parents' genes, and

Red Flag

If one of your parents was diagnosed with heart disease at age 55 or younger, you are at high risk for heart attack. It's important to be diligent about diet and exercise, and to regularly see a physician to have your blood pressure and cholesterol levels tested, regardless of your age or weight.

that combination may or may not cause you to develop atherosclerosis and coronary artery disease.

We all need to be aware of our family medical history. If one of your parents was diagnosed with heart disease at age 55 or younger, that's a red flag whether you're a son or a daughter. So you need to be diligent about diet and exercise, and regularly see a physician to have your blood pressure and cholesterol levels tested. Because of your genetics, your stakes are increased!

Even if heredity does increase your risk of developing heart disease, its severity could be less than that experienced by your parents. On the other hand, it could be worse. So, rather than letting your family's history of heart disease be an omen, just be aware of it when you and your physician discuss your medical examinations. This important exchange of information may result in closer surveillance of your health, including more frequent blood pressure and blood checks plus periodic heart stress testing.

Individuals with a family history of heart disease need to begin managing "modifiable" risk factors. You can't change your genetic makeup or your family history. But you *can* begin walking every day, cutting back on junk food, and eating more vegetables and grains. And you must educate yourself about high blood pressure and high cholesterol.

If you're overweight, aim for a more normal weight level, or at least lose *some* weight. Losing even a little weight produces positive results—it's the percentage of weight lost, rather than the number of pounds which counts. Diabetes also significantly increases your risk of heart disease and undesirable heart events, so it's crucial to be aware of and control your blood sugar levels.

You can make lifestyle changes that *absolutely* reduce your likelihood of developing heart disease. Remember, it's never too late to quit smoking, begin exercising, or improve your diet. However, don't wait until heart disease occurs before making key changes. The goal is to prevent heart disease from starting—or if it has started, to do everything possible to halt its progression—and to eliminate the likelihood of a heart attack.

Heart surgeons and cardiologists can do great things, but heart attacks permanently damage the heart, and that damage almost always leads to further problems. Not only are these problems costly in terms of treatment, lost workdays, and hindering physical and social activity, they also can be lethal.

Quick Quiz

Heart attacks can result in:

- (a) Damaged heart muscle
- (b) Leaky heart valves
- (c) Heart rhythm abnormalities
- (d) Congestive heart failure
- (e) Reduced exercise capacity
- (f) All of the above

Answer: **(f)** All of the above.

Does Heart Disease Only Strike Adults?

Thanks to research being performed at the Cleveland Clinic, we know that atherosclerosis—the gradual accumulation of plaque on the inside walls of arteries—can begin early in life.

Clinic researchers used a sophisticated imaging tool called intravascular ultrasound to examine donor hearts prior to transplantation. (In most cases, diagnostic angiograms where dye is injected directly into the heat arteries are performed to verify the suitability of the coronary arteries.) *Although many of the donated hearts came from adults in their 30s,* the study revealed the presence of atherosclerosis in the coronary arteries.

Early signs of atherosclerosis, such as fatty streaks, are showing up in the aorta (the body's biggest artery) of teenagers. Complicating the picture is the increased incidence of diabetes and obesity (a condition sometimes referred to as "diabesity") among children and adolescents. The diabetes that overweight children develop is type 2 diabetes, which for decades was seen mainly in adults. Type 2 diabetes is characterized by insulin resistance and the inability of the body's tissues to effectively utilize insulin.

Insulin is produced by the pancreas, which manages the body's blood sugar (glucose) levels. Insulin helps to transport the glucose provided by ingested food out of the bloodstream and into fat and muscle cells, which rely on glucose for energy. For unknown reasons, these cells can become resistant to insulin's effects. Over time, the cells don't get enough glucose and die, just as they can die from inadequate oxygen. Meanwhile, the glucose that isn't getting into fat and muscle cells accumulates in the bloodstream and over time creates horrendous problems for the body.

Without vigilant diabetes management, uncontrolled blood-glucose levels can damage nerves, organs, and eyes. In addition, diabetes and heart disease are often companions. This is a serious issue because diabetes can promote atherosclerosis and clot development in the arteries, as well as a condition called endothelial dysfunction, or abnormal reactivity of the blood vessels. In fact, a person with diabetes has a significantly greater chance for a heart attack.

Fortunately, the effects of type 2 diabetes and heart disease can be mitigated by weight reduction, regular exercise, an improved diet, and effective medications.

Am I Safe if My Weight Is Normal?

Unfortunately, being of normal weight or even thin doesn't eliminate your risks of heart attack or heart disease. People of all shapes and sizes have heart attacks and undiagnosed heart disease. Genes could very well account for our ability to stay slim, but they could also place us at high risk for heart attack.

Being a world-class athlete doesn't cut the risk either: in 1984, at age 52, long-distance runner Jim Fixx dropped dead from a heart attack during a workout. In 1995, champion Russian pairs skater Sergei Grinkov collapsed on the ice during a Monday morning practice. The two-time gold medalist was 28 years old. An autopsy confirmed advanced coronary artery blockages.

Being thin may give you an edge in reducing your risk of heart attack, but other factors can negate that benefit. For example, people who maintain proper weight, yet smoke, eat poorly, and don't exercise are still risking their health in a disproportionately adverse manner.

In fact, weight can be a poor indicator of what's going on inside our arteries—particularly in the coronary and carotid arteries, the latter supplying blood to the brain. These arteries are key targets for potentially lethal plaque accumulation. Other dangerous sites are inside the small blood vessels, where high blood pressure manifests itself. A person's weight does not signify what's going on inside the bloodstream, where good and bad cholesterol circulate, or within the cells, which can be damaged by inadequate glucose management due to diabetes.

Genes, diabetes, smoking, high cholesterol, and high blood pressure all increase our risks of heart disease and heart attack. So don't lower your guard just because your body weight is normal. Instead, capitalize on that advantage by taking steps to address any modifiable risk factors.

Is It True That Normal Cholesterol Levels Equal No Heart Risk?

This would be nice if it were true, but it isn't. Certainly, if you have comparatively low levels of low-density lipoprotein (LDL, the "bad" cholesterol), data suggest that your chances of heart attack are much lower than if you have high levels of LDL. But again, it depends on a constellation of risk factors, and cholesterol is just one of them.

• • • **Fast Fact** • • •

High-density lipoprotein (HDL, the "good cholesterol) is important too. The higher the better. Exercise and weight loss both improve HDL cholesterol. Unlike lowering LDL cholesterol with prescription medication, the impact of prescription medication on raising HDL cholesterol is less successful.

• • •

Don't More Men Get Heart Disease than Women?

This is only half true. Women most assuredly develop heart disease and have heart attacks; in fact, heart disease, not breast cancer, is the number one killer of women. Although women gain protection from heart disease from the hormone estrogen, they lose this protection with advancing age and after menopause. Actually, compared to men, heart attack increases significantly and faster among women around and after menopause. That's the time period when they catch up with men in terms of numbers.

Women who have a heart attack later in life fare much worse than men, even if they undergo protective interventions such as balloon angioplasty and stenting (the insertion of tiny cylindrical trusses that prop open an artery after it is cleared), or coronary artery bypass surgery. We don't know why, but those are the facts.

One of the problems is that there is less vigilance toward women with regard to screening and diagnosing heart disease. Even today, many physicians are not as alert or as aggressive as they should be about assessing women for heart disease. Also somewhat problematic is that symptoms such as exertional chest discomfort that clearly would be red flags for a possible heart attack in men are often discounted when they are seen in women. So, sometimes women aren't identified as being at high risk for developing heart disease.

But it's not just health care professionals who make this presumption; women themselves do it. Some women believe that they're simply not at risk for heart disease, even if they have symptoms. Such notions can delay investigation. Cardiologists have an obligation to educate women about heart disease, and physicians who care for adult women need to educate their patients about appropriate and safe care before, during, and after menopause.

Please Note

Campaigns for heart disease prevention in women are increasing. The Heart Truth campaign has made inroads in this regard. The bottom line: heart disease kills and it has no gender bias.

Hormone Therapy and Heart Disease

In February 2007, the American Heart Association updated its "Guidelines for Cardiovascular Disease Prevention in Women." In this publication, a leadership panel recommended that "providers should not use menopausal therapies such as hormone replacement therapy (HRT) or selective estrogen receptor modulators (SERMS) such as raloxifene or tamoxifene to prevent heart disease because they have been shown to be ineffective in protecting the heart and may increase the risk of stroke." In a February 2006 publication in the Archives of Internal Medicine, in close to 11,000 women who had previously undergone a hysterectomy, the authors concluded that "Conjugated equine estrogens provided no overall protection against myocardial infarction or coronary death in generally healthy postmenopausal women during a 7-year period of use. There was a suggestion of lower coronary heart disease risk with CEE among women 50 to 59 years of age at baseline." In the January 2006 *Journal of Women's Health,* Harvard researchers at Brigham and Women's Hospital reported that coronary heart disease was significantly reduced among Women's Health Initiative participants who began hormone therapy near menopause, as opposed to many years afterward—suggesting that the timing of hormone therapy determines whether it will help protect the heart. The best recommendation at present is that the decision to begin HRT is best individualized between the patient and her physician. Those patients who are experiencing symptoms of estrogen deficiency such as hot flashes can and do benefit from symptom relief. Until more is known, the indiscriminate prescription of HRT should be avoided.

I Thought Cigarettes and Cigars Affect the Lungs, Not the Heart?

Totally untrue. In addition to increasing the risks of lung, mouth, and other cancers, smoking raises blood pressure and promotes atherosclerosis—both of which are bad for the heart *and* blood vessels. Smokers may be familiar with the risks they take with regard to their lungs, but they need to know what smoking does to the blood vessels.

Smoking causes endothelial dysfunction (a kind of vessel paralysis) in the arteries. This means arteries are less able to widen to accommodate changes in blood flow and vessel pressure that occur in the body. The clinical name for this condition is impaired vasoreactivity, *vaso* meaning blood vessel and *reactivity* meaning the widening or contracting ability of the muscle within the wall of the artery. When blood vessels don't widen sufficiently, they can't help increase blood flow during periods of stress or strenuous physical activity. In fact, endothelial dysfunction *interferes* with adequate blood flow.

Endothelial dysfunction impedes the flow of red blood cells packed with oxygen for delivery to other cells, which will ensure their function and keep them alive. This includes the muscle cells of the heart, so that smokers are more susceptible to exercise-induced heart muscle dysfunction and are more likely to experience heart rhythm disturbances (see chapter 3). This problem can occur in the absence of coronary artery narrowing.

Smoking also damages the endothelial lining, the thin but crucial innermost layer of an artery wall that is in direct contact with the bloodstream. This damage promotes atherogenesis (formation of cholesterol plaque on the artery wall) and can accelerate the formation of brand new plaque and the progression of existing plaque.

I've Smoked This Long; Is There Any Point in Quitting Now?

It's never too late to quit smoking. Over time, depending on the age at which you quit, your cardiac risk begins to approach that of a nonsmoker. You also will reduce your risks of lung cancer and other cancers associated with smoking (bladder, mouth, breast, colon, and others). And if you're not smoking, you're not exposing people around you—your spouse, children, loved ones, and coworkers—to secondhand smoke, which also causes cancer and heart disease.

Does Using Cholesterol-Lowering Drugs Absolve Me from Keeping to a Healthy Diet?

No doubt about it—statins (the most widely prescribed cholesterol-lowering drugs) can cut your risk of cardiac events by lowering total and LDL (the "bad" cholesterol) levels, raising HDL (the "good" cholesterol) levels, and stabilizing and even reversing coronary artery disease. There's also evidence that statins help to shore up unstable plaque by reducing the likelihood that fatty deposits will fissure and render a coronary artery completely obstructed, causing a potentially fatal heart attack—or lead to further arterial narrowing as a clot forms to mend the break. These are all incredibly important and valuable cardiac benefits from one drug class.

But taking a statin isn't a green light for eating anything you want to eat or pulling the plug on your exercise regime. An irresponsible diet and lifestyle of inactivity can easily counteract the medication's beneficial effects. This is one of many scenarios in which patients must actively participate in their health care. Having a physician prescribe a cholesterol-lowering drug will do about 50 percent of the job in reducing your cholesterol level. But the other 50 percent has to come from you, the patient. That means:

- Educating yourself about your family history of heart disease.
- Learning and keeping track of your blood pressure and cholesterol levels.
- Quitting smoking.
- Adopting and maintaining a healthy diet.

- Engaging in an aerobic exercise program that keeps your heart rate elevated for at least thirty minutes continuously. Do this four to five times a week.

You should be taking a statin if you have prominent risk factors (such as elevated LDL cholesterol) for coronary artery disease or if you now have coronary artery disease. If you're at high risk, and your doctor hasn't put you on a statin medication, ask why, even if you have normal or near-normal cholesterol levels. Not only do statins help lower levels of bad cholesterol, they also can help stabilize plaque, which means they help reduce the risk of plaque rupture and heart attack.

• • • *Fast Fact* • • •

Even patients who are at a significant risk for coronary artery disease but have normal cholesterol can benefit from statins. This has recently been noted in patients with LDL cholesterol levels less than 130 mg/dl and elevated ultra sensitive C-reactive protein levels.

• • •

Statins possess side effects, such as myositis (muscle injury) and reversible liver dysfunction, but both of these are manageable and occur in a very small percentage of patients. Typically, three months after beginning a statin medication, return to your physician for follow-up and blood tests to rule out the presence of myositis or liver problems. If everything checks out satisfactorily, then return for similar follow-ups every six months.

The most common reasons patients quit statins are perceived muscle aches or gastrointestinal upset. But such side effects are comparatively rare, occurring in less than 5 percent of the millions of people in the U.S. and abroad taking statins. With proper monitoring, that risk will be far outweighed by the known benefits. Focusing on potential side effects and deciding not to take a statin can be a shortsighted decision. These medications have been actively prescribed for twenty-plus years, are one of the most thoroughly researched classes of medications, and have been proven to reduce the incidence of heart attacks, strokes, and vascular death in countless studies. If you are at risk or have been diagnosed with coronary artery disease and your physician does not suggest a statin, ask why!

Are Heart Attacks Caused by "Clogged Pipes"?

Until several years ago, heart attack was generally interpreted as the result of a gradual accumulation of plaque that eventually narrows an artery so severely that blood flow is nearly or completely cut off. This was sometimes referred to as the "clogged pipes" model, the analogy being that a coronary artery is much like a drainpipe whose inner wall accumulates so much corrosion and debris that blood flow all but stops. And when blood flow ceases, a heart attack occurs.

We now know that was a vast oversimplification. It's true that, over time, plaque accumulation inside an artery wall can progress to the point where it impedes blood flow and produces chest pain, the classic symptom of heart disease and heart attack. That does occur, but in the minority of heart attack cases.

The real heart attack culprit is unstable, soft plaque that accumulates on arterial walls. It's called unstable plaque because it develops cracks easily. A tiny fissure can develop in the plaque, and when that happens, the body's normal mechanism for dealing with such tissue injury—blood clot (thrombus) formation—kicks into action. Clot formation in a narrowing artery is a dangerous event. The clot can quickly swell in size and severely restrict or block blood flow, causing a heart attack.

Also, unstable plaque is typically found in arteries that exhibit only slight or moderate narrowing. So, traditional imaging tools can provide a rather limited or misleading picture of the seriousness of the problem. In other words, mild or moderate coronary disease may not appear on standard EKG (electrocardiography) testing or through stress tests, but you still may be at risk of heart attack due to plaque rupture in the near future that at present is difficult to predict.

Do I Have to Follow an Extreme Exercise Routine to Protect Myself Against Heart Disease?

Many people are apprehensive about exercise because they think the only way they'll benefit from it is by training like Olympic athletes. But that assumption couldn't be further from the truth.

With exercise, it's not the intensity that's important; it's the quality, duration, and in my view, most importantly, the regularity. Very beneficial results can come from thirty minutes of quality exercise, performed four to five days a week. Here are some examples of aerobic exercise:

- Jogging or running
- Swimming
- Jumping rope
- Aerobic classes
- Yoga
- Pilates
- Tennis
- Ice skating, rollerblading
- Cycling, spinning
- Brisk walking

Additional Info

I recommend my patients aim for thirty minutes of aerobic exercise seven days per week. Since life is unpredictable, if you take this approach, you should be able to exercise at least five days per week. Exercise should be considered as important as eating, sleeping, and personal hygiene. Put it on your "must do" list.

The following weight-bearing exercises are also beneficial because they help maintain bone mass:

- Walking, running, or hiking
- Lifting weights
- Using a treadmill or elliptical machine
- Rock climbing
- Jumping rope
- Skiing

Although the ideal exercise regimen is seven days a week, the most important factor people should remember is that some exercise is better than no exercise. Any exercise that gets you moving on a consistent basis—and safely raises the heart rate for a sustained period—is beneficial. (For more details regarding exercise, see chapter 9.)

Can Minor Changes in Diet Still Help Reduce Heart Attack Risk?

The most heart-friendly diets are low in cholesterol and saturated fat. Strict vegetarian, plant-based, zero-fat diets are admirable, healthy choices. But for most of us, such a diet is unrealistic and may be unsatisfying. Yet there are many easy ways to improve a diet without purging it of foods you enjoy, and as with exercise, some change is better than none at all.

Your approach to diet modification should be similar to launching an exercise program: choose a healthy diet that you can maintain. If you choose unrealistic goals for your new eating habits, you set yourself up for frustration and failure. If you set realistic goals, you'll achieve them and be inspired to stick with the program.

Your new diet should simply be healthier than what it is currently. If your new diet is 50 percent healthier, that's 50 percent better than no change whatsoever. So start with incremental yet meaningful improvements, and over time cut back on these "bad guys":

- Fast food
- Fried food
- Junk food
- Processed food
- Soda pop
- Alcohol (yes, it's fattening)
- Deli sandwiches
- Bagels, muffins, and breakfast pastries
- Creamy salad dressings
- Energy bars and drinks
- Ice cream
- Donuts, cookies, and cakes
- Lattes and mochas

At the same time, reintroduce—or perhaps introduce—your taste buds and digestive system to vegetables, grains, brown rice, fruits, and steamed, baked, or broiled (not fried) fish.

How Does Stress Affect Heart Disease?

Stress has its place in life; it keeps us alert in the face of danger, helps us meet deadlines, and makes us more focused at work. But chronic, unmanaged stress is bad for the heart.

Unlike traditional risk factors (high cholesterol, high blood pressure, a sedentary lifestyle), stress is tough to measure. We do know that stress raises blood pressure and has a negative impact on blood-vessel function in the same way smoking does. If you have unavoidable stress in your life, exercise can play a great role in stress reduction. Certainly, any activity that you enjoy and that takes your mind away from stress can also be beneficial.

Consider these stress-busting activities:

- Fishing
- Reading
- Watching a great movie
- Getting a massage
- Meditating
- Practicing yoga
- Spending quality time with family or friends

Indeed, the best stress management program combines exercise with one or more of these activities.

Chapter 2

Your Heart's Anatomy

N ow that we've explored some common questions and myths about heart health, let's take a closer look at this wonderful, dynamic organ.

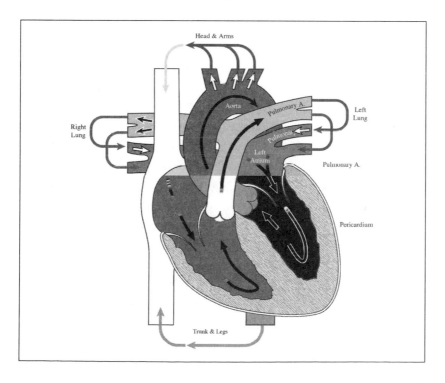

The heart is a collection of blood vessels (arteries and veins), chambers, valves, and electrical nodes and fibers, all built in and around three layers of special muscle tissue. The outermost layer of heart muscle is the epicardium. The coronary arteries, which are visible on the epicardium, distribute oxygen-rich blood throughout the heart tissue. The epicardium covers the myocardium, and the endocardium—the inner surface of the heart—is in direct contact with blood.

The heart has four cardiac chambers: two upper and two lower. During each contraction/relaxation cycle, blood flows into and out of the chambers. The upper cardiac chambers (atria) receive blood, while the lower chambers (ventricles) pump blood into the body. Each chamber contains a valve that manages the blood flowing into and out of the chamber and big vessels. These valves ensure that blood flows freely in a forward direction and, under normal circumstances, prevent unwanted backflow (leakage) of blood into the chambers. Blood in the heart's chambers is constantly moving, ensuring the adequate delivery of oxygen to the body's tissues, sustaining life.

Without electrical stimulation, the heart can't contract and therefore can't pump. The electrical nodes and fibers run the heart's electrical conduction system, the nucleus of which is the heart's own internal pacemaker—the one that we are all born with, the sinoatrial node.

An easy way to understand basic heart anatomy and function involves breaking everything down into four functional areas:

- Plumbing
- Electricity
- Muscle
- Valves

Plumbing: Cardiovascular System Basics

Before reviewing the plumbing within the heart, let's take a quick look at the overall plumbing of the cardiovascular system—the heart and the blood vessels that spread throughout the body. The cardiovascular system has two types of vessels: those that carry blood away from the heart and those that return blood to it. Both types of blood vessels begin and end their journeys through the body at the heart.

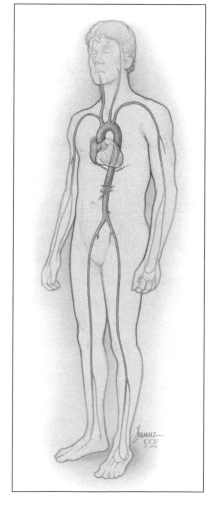

Red blood cells with freshly received lung oxygen travel away from the heart to the rest of the body in arteries, which form the arterial system. After red blood cells deliver their oxygen to the tissues, the deoxygenated red blood cells are routed back to the heart in veins, which form the venous system. Once back in the heart, the deoxygenated blood is pumped by the right ventricle into the lungs, then via the left atrium to the left ventricle, then out through the aorta, the body's largest blood vessel and the gateway to the arterial system.

Are Arteries and Veins Connected?

The entire cardiovascular system is a "closed" loop, meaning that at points throughout the body, all arteries are connected to all veins. In

Did You Know?

The blood vessels comprise thousands of miles throughout the body. At the level of the smallest blood vessel (capillary), oxygen leaves the blood cell and is transferred (diffused) across the capillary wall to the awaiting tissue. This occurs because there is a higher oxygen concentration in the blood vessel compared to the awaiting tissue. This is termed an oxygen gradient and serves as a signal for the needed oxygen transfer.

other words, everywhere the arterial system courses through the body, so too does the venous system, because blood that leaves the heart must eventually return to it.

The largest vessels of the arterial system originate in the heart, and the largest vessels of the venous system end there. As both systems fan out from the heart, multiple branchings occur, just as rivers branch off into tributaries, streams, and creeks.

At myriad points throughout the body, the vessels of both systems grow progressively more slender, until they branch off into capillaries, the tiny collection of vessels that connect both the arterial and venous systems. Capillaries are so narrow that red blood cells move through them in single file. Capillaries close the loop, permitting constant recirculation of blood throughout the body.

The amount of blood in the human body, or blood volume, is governed by body surface area, so different-sized people have different amounts of blood. (Altitude also can affect blood volume; people living in higher altitudes tend to have a greater blood volume than those living at lower altitudes.)

On average, however, an adult weighing 150 to 160 pounds has approximately five quarts of blood (5 liters, 1.3 U.S. gallons, or 10.5 U.S. pints). If a person is at rest, the blood travels around the body and back to the heart in about one minute. The heart beats seventy times a minute; with each beat, the heart pumps 60 to 90 milliliters (2 to 3 ounces) of blood out of the heart. It can move 5 to 7 liters of blood in one minute and 7,600 liters (2,000 gallons) per day. Over the course of a lifetime, it beats more than 2.5 billion times and pumps more than 200 million liters of blood. Given these numbers, it is truly an incredible organ, highlighting the importance of preserving its optimal function.

• • • *Fast Fact* • • •

Checking your pulse can be tricky. I usually demonstrate to my patients how to correctly check their pulse. You need to familiarize yourself with the location of the radial artery, which is one of two main arteries feeding your arm beginning at your elbows and ending at your wrists. The radial artery is located on the thumb side portion of your wrist when your palm is facing upward toward the ceiling.

With your palm facing upward, use your opposite first and second fingers to reach over and *lightly* feel for your pulse on the opposite wrist. If you press too hard, you may not feel your pulse, instead compressing it. I would encourage you to use variable amounts of pressure, starting out lightly and increasing until you detect your pulse. Once you have located your radial pulse and determined its cadence (hopefully regular!), simultaneously look at a clock or watch with a second hand. Count the number of pulsations that you detect at your wrist over a fifteen-second period and multiply by four. That is your pulse rate. You might consider repeating this a few times to ensure accuracy.

• • •

What Makes Up the Heart's Plumbing?

We're born with two major heart arteries: the left and the right main coronary arteries. These vessels are the heart's main conduits. With their ever-narrowing branches, they help route oxygenated blood over the heart's exterior and then arborize (branch out like trees) beneath the heart's surface to ensure that all the cells of the heart are nourished.

The left main coronary artery splits early into the left anterior descending (LAD) and left circumflex coronary arteries. Saying that a vessel divides "early" simply means that it doesn't travel far before branching occurs; the left main coronary artery, for instance, is less than one inch in length. Of course, the entire cardiovascular system is a massive series of branching vessels. "Later" segments are progressively narrower.

The LAD coronary artery traverses the front of the heart, while the left circumflex coronary artery courses across the side and sometimes the back of the heart. The right coronary artery lies predominantly on the back of the heart. These major coronary arteries each serve roughly one-third of the heart muscle, and they provide a balanced and efficient delivery of oxygenated blood.

• • • *Fast Fact* • • •

Occasionally, a patient is born with abnormal coronary arteries. What I mean is a congenital abnormality exists where a coronary artery arises from an abnormal location, is exceedingly small, or just plain does not exist. Fortunately, these occurrences are quite rare, are most commonly found incidentally, and generally do not impact the patient.

• • •

Keep in mind that there is normal variation in anatomy from one person to the next. Anatomical illustrations like those in this chapter are just representations of the norm. Everyone is a little different. Sometimes the right coronary artery is larger and the left circumflex is smaller, or vice versa. Such natural anatomic variables are part of what makes each of us unique.

What Happens if the Pipes—the Blood Vessels— Get Clogged?

As we discussed earlier, arteries—particularly the coronary arteries—are prone to plaque accumulation, or atherosclerosis. If the accumulated plaque is unstable, a fissure can develop and set the stage for vessel blockage (occlusion) that can abruptly halt blood

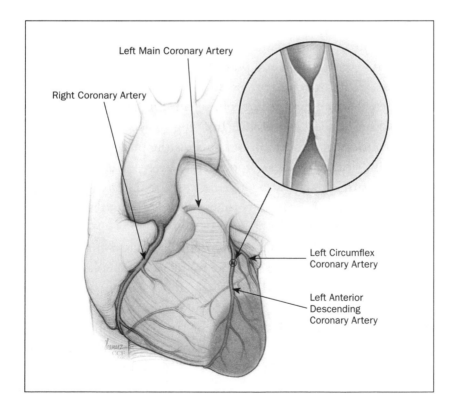

Left Main Coronary Artery

Right Coronary Artery

Left Circumflex
Coronary Artery

Left Anterior
Descending
Coronary Artery

flow. When blood flow slows down or stops altogether, the heart muscle quickly becomes starved for oxygen. Heart muscle tissue cells cry out in agony, which we may experience as chest discomfort. If, after a few minutes coronary artery blood flow remains obstructed, heart muscle cells die, irreversibly losing their pumping function, and a heart scar forms.

This is a heart attack.

Such blockages can occur anywhere within the three major coronary arteries. Heart tissue lying just beyond the blockage is at significant risk for damage. A full blockage (100 percent occlusion) that develops "early on" in a coronary artery causes a significant heart attack, because oxygenated blood can't get to a substantial portion of heart muscle downstream from the blockage.

Conversely, if the blockage occurs in the terminal aspect of a coronary artery (a comparatively narrow section near its end) or in a very narrow side branch, a heart attack will damage a smaller portion of heart muscle tissue. Sometimes the area of damage is so small that heart function and pumping capacity are imperceptibly changed and are therefore preserved.

When a heart attack occurs, physicians must locate and relieve the blockage as soon as possible. Imaging tools such as x-ray and catheterization, and interventions such as the placement of stents (tiny cylindrical trusses that prop open an artery after it is cleared) or bypass surgery (rerouting the heart's circulation to improve arterial blood flow) focus on coronary arteries that are epicardial, coursing the surface of the heart.

But these vessels also take important downward turns, diving into the heart tissue itself to serve the middle and inner layers of the heart with oxygenated blood. As they do, they become progressively narrower, until they're just microns wide (microscopic in size), so they can provide oxygen and nutrients to individual heart cells. [The portions of vessels that are intramyocardial (within the myocardium) lie below the surface, within the heart muscle itself.]

The main focus of coronary artery intervention is on the epicardial segments of arteries, which are the larger conduits or plumbing pipes. And thus far, this focus has been effective in managing coronary artery disease.

However, current imaging tools don't provide the clarity needed to detect significant blockages in the intramyocardial arteries, except for segments just below the heart's surface. But if you have atherosclerosis and narrowing of your epicardial arteries, you will have the same problem in your intramyocardial arteries, because atherosclerosis is a diffuse disease. It doesn't occur only at one location or in one vessel. It affects arteries throughout the heart and body to varying degrees.

• • • *Fast Fact* • • •

Atherosclerosis is systemic, meaning it can be found throughout all of the arteries within the body. That is why it's so important to modify your risk factors. For example, blockages occur in the arteries leading to the kidneys, negatively impacting kidney function and contributing to high blood pressure, ultimately leading to the enhanced occurrence of stroke and heart attack.

Other common areas for atherosclerotic deposits include the carotid arteries leading to the brain, the abdominal aorta—the main pipe serving the abdominal organs—and the arteries leading to the legs and feet.

It is in our human nature not to think about this sort of thing on a daily basis. And I agree—it should not be on your mind. Instead focusing on a healthy lifestyle and following up with your physician for periodic checkups are important.

• • •

Not having "access" to these very narrow vessels below the heart's surface is a bit limiting. That's why medication and risk-factor modification, such as diet and exercise, play important roles in heart health management.

• • • *Fast Fact* • • •

Using cholesterol-lowering agents such as statins helps to manage systemic atherosclerosis, stabilizing it and, ideally, partially reversing it.

• • •

Electricity: The Heart's Conduction System

Just as the heart would be a meaningless mass of tissue without a constant source of blood, it would be an idle pump without a constant

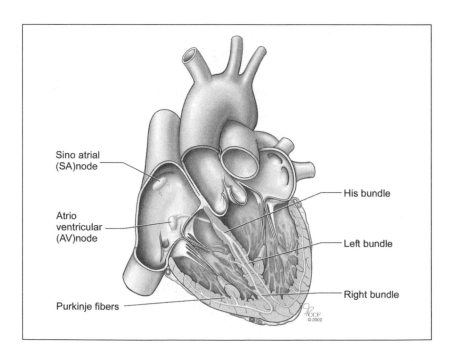

Sino atrial (SA)node

His bundle

Atrio ventricular (AV)node

Left bundle

Right bundle

Purkinje fibers

CCF
© 2002

source of electrical stimulation. That crucial stimulation and its conduction throughout the heart's tissue stem from special collections of "pacemaker" cells strategically located throughout the heart:

- The sinoatrial node (SAN), located in the upper portion of the right atrial wall, just below the entrance to the superior vena cava (the large vein that carries deoxygenated blood from the head, neck, arms, and chest to the heart)

- The atrial-ventricular node (AVN), located in the lower portion of the interatrial septum, the wall of tissue that separates the heart's upper chambers

- The His-Purkinje system, a series of muscle fibers and "bundles" that course throughout the heart chamber walls

These three components represent a vital portion of the heart's electrical conduction system, which is responsible for discharging electrical impulses throughout the cardiac tissue. This electrical excitation governs the constant contraction and relaxation of the heart's upper and lower chambers.

The heart's electrical system begins its work as we develop in the womb and continues until our last breath. Normally, in healthy humans, the heart's conduction system fires 60 to 100 impulses every minute, every day.

Please Note

The above pacemaker centers are ones we are all born with. Do not confuse these specialized electrical tissue centers with an artificial pacemaker, which is a battery pack with wires, placed inside the body when the heart's electrical system fails to maintain a sufficient heart rate and forward blood pumping.

Red Flag

Should you notice a reduction in your pulse rate, especially if associated with a lack of energy, shortness of breath, or light-headedness and near fainting, this could be an indicator of a faulty cardiac electrical system. For example, if your heart rate over a period of years averaged 70 beats per minute, and you now check your pulse at your wrist and record a pulse rate of 30 beats per minute, this is a significant change. For these symptoms to develop solely because of a low heart rate, the decrease in the pulse must be significant. A change of a few beats per minute is not of any consequence.

How Does the Heart Keep Pumping?

The heart's pacemaker cells (also called neural cells) are very different from muscle cells in that they cannot contract. What they do possess—and this makes them unique in the body—is "intrinsic automaticity." Basically, under normal circumstances, pacemaker cells emit between approximately 60 and 100 electrical impulses per minute to drive heart contractions. In a way, this conduction system is the "nervous system" of the heart, controlling heartbeats and ensuring constant, adequate blood circulation.

In a normal, healthy heart, cardiac impulses originate from the SAN, the heart's natural internal pacemaker. SAN cells generate electrical impulses that travel through a fine network of electrical interconnections embedded in tissue throughout the heart walls and muscle.

This impulse spreads first through the heart's upper chambers and then, with help from the AVN, to its lower chambers. Electrical activation of the lower chambers generates a contraction of the cardiac muscle cells in unison, creating the main coordinated pumping action of the ventricles.

The resulting heartbeat represents the coordinated ejection of deoxygenated blood from the right ventricle into the pulmonary artery, which sends the blood to the lungs for reoxygenation, and the ejection of oxygenated blood from the left ventricle into the aorta, which then sends that blood throughout the body. A contraction spreads nearly instantaneously across the heart in milliseconds (thousandths of a second).

How Does Aging Affect the Heart?

Just as with other tissues and organs in our bodies, the function of the conduction system can deteriorate over time, and the otherwise smooth activation of impulses and systematic spread of the conduction wave through the atria and ventricles become less coordinated.

Our systems at age 75 may not transmit electrical impulses with the rapidity and coordination that they did at age 35. There are several possible causes:

- A natural decline in the number of SAN cells
- Fat accumulation around the cells
- Medications that depress cardiac electrical function
- Viral infections
- Exposure of the heart to toxins, such as excessive amounts of alcohol
- A heart attack that scars the tissue lying near the electrical conduction system
- Prior cardiac surgery
- Valvular heart disease

Pacemaker cells, like other tissue cells in the body, depend on a constant blood supply. Impairing that supply can cause parts of our heart's electrical system to short-circuit, which can lead to uncoordinated electrical activity, slow heart rates, and reduced heart blood output. Common symptoms in such cases include shortness of breath, fatigue, lightheadedness, and even fainting. If symptoms do not subside, patients may need to undergo surgical implantation of a pacemaker. (For more about conduction problems that also can cause cardiac rhythm disturbances, see chapter 3.)

Here's one thing to keep in mind: not everyone diagnosed with a conduction system condition needs a man-made pacemaker. That's because, in addition to working with the SAN, the heart conduction system's other components can serve as backup pacemakers if function is impaired. In other words, nature provides a built-in backup. Pacemaker implantation should be an individual and carefully considered decision made by you and your physician.

In addition, cardiac conditions that cause abnormal enlargement of the heart, such as heart failure, can irritate the electrical conduction system and increase the likelihood of heart-rhythm disturbances, which can be dangerous and life threatening. And a heart attack can cause heart-tissue scarring, which might lead to the development of abnormal heart rhythms.

• • • *Fast Fact* • • •

The majority of heart disease deaths are secondary to an abnormal heart rhythm disturbance originating from the bottom chambers (ventricles) of the heart. Coronary artery blockage and heart attack raise the likelihood of this occurrence significantly. Many of these sudden electrical occurrences, termed sudden cardiac death, occur at home during the acute heart attack phase before a patient reaches the attention of healthcare professionals. For this reason, automatic external defibrillators (AEDs) are now more prevalent in public areas including shopping malls and airports, where a high concentration of people can be found.

• • •

Muscle: Sheer Strength

The heart is perhaps the most durable and reliable muscle in the body. The special cardiac cells that compose that muscle work in unison to produce an amazing 100,000 heartbeats per day without interruption and without voluntary coaxing.

But, like other muscles, the heart can become fatigued if it's asked to do too much. For instance, uncontrolled high blood pressure can contribute to the development of atherosclerosis, which, as we know, can impede normal blood flow. High blood pressure can also cause different types of cardiomyopathy, which affects heart muscle.

In cardiomyopathy, one or more of the heart's chambers may become enlarged (dilated), with abnormally thin walls; alternatively the heart muscle may thicken, or the heart muscle may become rigid. Each of these problems can weaken the heart's pumping action and lead to heart failure because the heart is unable to consistently pump enough blood out to the body to keep cells nourished, oxygenated, and healthy.

In heart failure, blood and fluid pool in the lungs and accumulate in the feet, ankles, and legs. People with heart failure experience significant fatigue and shortness of breath. Heart failure is

Did You Know?

Cardiomyopathy is derived from the prefix cardio, meaning *heart,* and the suffix *myopathy,* meaning abnormally functioning muscle. In fact, medical terms are combinations of suffixes and prefixes. Once mastered, this terminology can be extremely helpful in comprehending medical reports and communicating with your physician.

often a long, slow, costly, debilitating, and demoralizing condition that can shorten the lives of those afflicted.

How Do Hypertension and Heart Attack Affect the Heart?

Even when arteries are healthy, abnormally high blood pressure (hypertension) can cause severe problems. High blood pressure can interfere with blood flow from the heart's surface to the inner layers of muscle lying below. The pressure increases the gradient for blood flow; in a sense, blood now has to push "uphill." This increase also raises risks of heart attack, stroke, heart rhythm disturbances, and congestive heart failure due to the added stress and strain on the cardiac muscle.

Another possible cause of abnormally high blood pressure inside the heart is aortic stenosis, a valvular heart problem that severely restricts ejection of blood from the left ventricle, the main pumping chamber. Also, in conditions such as anemia, where a long-term reduction in the red blood cell count decreases the oxygen-carrying capacity of the blood, the heart attempts to compensate by pumping with greater vigor. Over time, without intervention, the heart muscle becomes fatigued and weakens.

A heart attack also can permanently damage valuable heart muscle by increasing the pumping burden for the remaining non-damaged and therefore normal tissue. For example, if one-third of the heart's muscle tissue became nonfunctional due to scarring from a heart attack, the remaining two-thirds would have to work harder to maintain an equivalent output of blood. You can imagine that over time this places an increasing burden on the heart and can lead to heart failure.

After a heart attack, the "architecture" of the heart undergoes a process called remodeling. The remaining normal heart muscle begins to contract too much (becoming "hypercontractile"), to compensate for the scarred and dysfunctional heart muscle. As this

Additional Info

Heart remodeling can be favorably affected through the use of heart medications. It is important to discuss the role of medication with your physician to ensure your satisfactory recovery after a heart attack.

hypercontractile state persists, the heart muscle begins to enlarge, which in turn stretches and thins the heart chamber walls. Thinning in turn weakens the heart muscle, so that pumping ability gradually worsens.

This can become an unrelenting vicious cycle in which the initial heart attack causes heart enlargement, which leads to further heart enlargement. The result can be congestive heart failure.

Weakened, nonfunctional scar tissue in the heart is also potentially problematic because it's prone to aneurysm, an unwanted ballooning or "out-pouching" of the tissue. With aneurysm comes an increased risk for congestive heart failure and blood-clot formation in the heart. If a clot dislodges, that can mean major trouble if it travels through the artery (arterial embolism). Potential complications include stroke, heart-rhythm disturbances, and death.

What Separates the Different Parts of the Heart Muscle?

The right and left upper chambers of the heart are separated by a wall of tissue called the interatrial septum. Under normal circumstances, no "communication" occurs between the two atria. That's because the interatrial septum prevents the mixing of the deoxygenated blood on the right with the fully oxygenated blood on the left. The interatrial septum plays no role in heart contraction and is not subject to damage from a heart attack.

The interventricular septum is a thicker and more muscular wall that separates the heart's lower pumping chambers. In fact, it's one of the thickest structures inside the heart, composed of cardiac muscle cells. The interventricular septum possesses an abundant blood supply and actively participates in the contraction of both ventricles. Because it draws its blood supply from the coronary arteries, its tissue is susceptible to damage from a heart attack.

Valves

Let's take a closer look at the four valves of the heart. They are the right and left atrioventricular valves (AV valves) and the aortic and pulmonary valves (semilunar valves).

The right AV valve commonly is called the tricuspid valve; the left AV valve is known as the mitral valve. These valves are "atrioventricular" because they are each situated between an upper (atrial) and lower (ventricular) heart chamber and control the flow of blood pumped into a ventricle.

The aortic and pulmonary valves, respectively, control blood flow pumped out of the left and right ventricle and into major blood vessels.

Each valve is formed of special leaflets (flaps derived from cardiac tissue) that help control the intake or discharge of blood from the upper to lower chambers, or from the lower chambers out to the lungs and aorta. The valves help maintain proper blood-flow direction and, when closed, prevent unwanted backflow. The tricuspid valve is composed of three flaps, as are the aortic and pulmonary valves. The mitral valve is made up of two flaps.

The following table describes the locations and functions of the four valves.

Valves of the Heart	Location	Function
Tricuspid	On the right side of the heart, situated between the right atrium and right ventricle (right upper and lower heart chambers).	Controls flow of deoxygenated blood from the top chamber (right atrium) into the bottom chamber (right ventricle). From throughout the body, the deoxygenated blood enters the right atrium via the vena cavae, the body's largest veins. Veins return blood to the heart.
Pulmonary (also pulmonic)	On the right side of the heart, situated between the right ventricle (right lower chamber) and the pulmonary artery.	Controls flow of deoxygenated blood (pumped from the right ventricle) to the pulmonary artery, a large vessel that branches off to the lungs. Blood is sent to the lungs for reoxygenation.
Mitral	On the left side of the heart, situated between the left atrium and left ventricle (left upper and lower heart chambers).	Controls flow of blood from the top chamber (left atrium) into the bottom chamber (left ventricle). This is oxygenated blood sent directly from the lungs via the pulmonary veins.
Aortic	On the left side of the heart, situated between the left ventricle (left lower chamber) and the aorta.	Controls flow of oxygenated blood (pumped from the left ventricle) to the aorta, the body's main and largest artery. Arteries send blood away from the heart.

The tricuspid valve works in tandem with the pulmonary valve on the right side of the heart, and the mitral valve works in tandem with the aortic valve on the left side of the heart. The heart has a relaxation phase (diastole) and a contraction phase (systole). When the AV valves are open during diastole, the aortic and pulmonary valves are closed. When the heart contracts during systole, the aortic and pulmonary valves are open, and the mitral and tricuspid valves are closed.

How Do the AV Valves Work?

The tricuspid and mitral valves derive their function from an intricate system of collagen cords called chordae tendineae. These parachute-like strands anchor the valve cusps to the special papillary muscles, which protrude from the ventricular walls. The papillary muscles contract and relax in concert with pumping of the heart, greatly assisting the opening and closing of the valves.

This anchoring system is essential for proper valve function, particularly during ventricular contraction when the AV valves close. This action prevents blood from leaking backward into the upper heart chambers (right and left atria).

When the heart is relaxed and its chambers are filling with blood in anticipation of the next heartbeat or cardiac cycle, the AV valves are open. When the heart contracts, the AV valves close and blood is forced out of the ventricles: on the right, through the pulmonary valve and into the pulmonary arteries, which lead to the lungs; and on the left, through the aortic valve and into the aorta, the gateway to the arterial system. When the AV valves function well, sufficient blood passes through them when they are open, and no blood passes through them when they are closed.

However, certain cardiac diseases can undermine valve function, causing one of two problems. Stenosis restricts the valve's ability to open fully during the relaxation phase, while regurgitation, or leaking, results from incomplete valve closure during the contraction phase.

How Does a Heart Attack Affect the Valves?

Mitral regurgitation can be related to a heart attack. A heart attack can cause irreversible tissue damage to one or both papillary muscles, which are attached to the inner ventricular wall surface. Scarring in this area reduces the contractile and relaxation properties of the papillary muscles and impedes valve function. The papillary muscles shorten and stiffen, reducing the range of mitral valve leaflet motion. The valve can open reasonably well, but it cannot fully close during heart contraction, and the flaps can leak significantly.

Another source of mitral valve leakage is enlargement of the left ventricle due to scarring caused by a heart attack. This development causes enlargement of the mitral valve annulus, the ring-like support structure on which the valve is situated. Distortion of the annulus stretches the leaflets apart, preventing proper closure during contraction. This problem is called annular dilatation, and it causes valve leakage during contraction.

Mitral valve leakage results in both normal forward blood flow and abnormal backward blood flow on the left side of the heart—an extremely inefficient development. Severe leakage can cause an abnormal volume of blood in the ventricle, or volume overload, which over time leads to unwanted stretching, enlargement, and further weakening of the heart muscle. Unless we interrupt that

Please Note

Not all heart attacks affect mitral valve function. It depends on the location and size of the heart attack. This is not possible to predict. Medications administered during and after a heart attack can limit the size of heart damage and prevent adverse remodeling of the heart muscle, reducing the likelihood of significant mitral valve leakage.

cycle with mitral valve surgery, it's a downward spiral for the patient because it can lead to heart failure.

Checking Mitral Valve Function. Possible structural damage from a heart attack is one reason it's so important for physicians to listen to (auscultate) the heart on a regular basis. This is particularly important during acute hospitalization, when the first sounds of a developing mitral valve problem can be detected. Signs of a mitral valve problem may also be inaudible due to ambient noise in the hospital room. These are best assessed by a cardiac ultrasound test called an echocardiogram.

The sensitivity of today's echocardiography equipment allows for the detection of extremely mild mitral regurgitation. But the mere presence of leakage does not warrant surgical correction. In most cases, mild to moderate mitral valve leakage causes no symptoms and no long-term adverse consequences. Many times, mild mitral regurgitation can remain stable for decades without either surgery or medication. The physician and patient should carefully discuss echocardiography findings, and surgical intervention should not be suggested unless such a measure will benefit the patient and outweigh the surgical risk.

By contrast, patients with severe mitral valve leakage, particularly in the presence of heart dysfunction (such as heart attack), are at high risk for heart failure and death. The most common symptoms arising from severe mitral valve leakage are shortness of breath and fatigue, due to abnormally elevated pressures and fluid engorgement in the lungs. Mitral valve surgical intervention should be considered in these cases.

It's important to remember that, overall, only a small percentage of patients who have mitral valve leakage will truly need mitral valve surgery.

Chapter 3

What Is a Heart Attack?

Several terms are used to characterize heart attack severity. Unfortunately, some of them are misleading. These terms aren't used just by lay people, but also by the media and even physicians. For instance, sometimes an individual is described as having suffered a "mild" or "small" heart attack.

In truth, no heart attack is small or mild.

Heart attack is a diagnosis of damage to cardiac muscle—damage that can compromise heart function and lead to big problems down the road, including further heart attacks. Once you have a heart attack, regardless of its "size," your health prognosis is worse than if you had never experienced one.

That is why it is so important to modify your lifestyle to preempt future heart damage. If you experience symptoms of chest discomfort that were not present previously, seek prompt medical advice. You may well have coronary artery blockage and be experiencing symptoms that represent a prelude to heart attack. Not all symptoms emanating from the heart reflect actual damage. Symptoms that are periodic and associated, for example, with activity and relieved with rest are so-called warning signs of coronary arterial insufficiency. In this circumstance, if blockage is found and relieved either by stenting or bypass surgery, and consequently normal heart function is preserved, your prognosis is greatly improved compared to a patient who actually experiences heart damage. This is an important distinction that should be emphasized. Normal heart muscle is always better than weakened or abnormal heart muscle, irrespective of cause. For instance, irreversible heart muscle weakening due to a virus with normal coronary arteries devoid of blockage portends a worse prognosis compared to a patient with severe coronary artery disease, multiple successful coronary artery bypass grafts, and normal heart function.

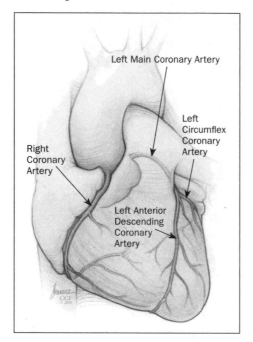

So when the terms *small* or *mild* get bandied about, particularly by physicians, what they're referring to is the extent of tissue damage caused by heart attack, as well as the level of enzyme leak.

Normal myocytes (healthy heart muscle cells) contain, among other things, a class of proteins found in no other cells in the body. If the protective membrane of a myocyte is damaged because it's starved for oxygen, those proteins can leach through the membrane and circulate in the bloodstream. After a heart attack, myocyte enzyme levels help determine the extent of cardiac tissue damage.

Small or mild heart attacks are those that, compared with "big" or "severe" heart attacks, cause comparatively little damage to heart tissue. In this book, heart attacks are characterized as small, medium/moderate, or large in terms of the damage they've caused to the heart muscle.

Although small heart attacks can cause symptoms just as noticeable and unsettling as those caused by a big heart attack, small events are less apt to result in the consequences associated with large heart attacks, such as heart failure, valve problems, and rhythm disturbances. But it's important to remember that we can't always equate heart attack severity with symptom severity. A "large" heart attack can cause "small" symptoms and vice versa.

• • • *Fast Fact* • • •

Just because your doctor tells you your heart attack was mild and you escaped the "big one" does not equate with complacency. You have now been diagnosed with coronary artery disease and your heart muscle has been damaged. This is serious business, necessitating the implementation of a sustained lifestyle modification program.

• • •

New Insights Into Coronary Artery Plaque

Most medical centers have the expertise to identify coronary artery narrowing, and patients with that condition are typically treated with a combination of interventions: bypass surgery, implantation of stents, and medical therapy.

In the wake of an intervention, patients may believe "I was a heart attack waiting to happen" and feel that such intervention eliminated all risk of heart attack. But they'd be mistaken. And one hopes their cardiologists would set them straight because the significance of plaque accumulation can be inappropriately minimized.

Until several years ago, it was believed that most heart attacks resulted from the progressive accumulation of plaque lining the inside wall of a coronary artery. As plaque accumulation increases, the theory went, the channel through which blood courses in the vessel (the lumen) begins to narrow.

Like corrosion on the inside of an old water pipe, the plaque builds and builds until it literally blocks the entire lumen. Within minutes of the blood supply being cut off for good, heart muscle cells fed by that coronary artery begin to die because they're receiving no oxygen (an event called myocardial infarction). And the person who owns those arteries experiences a heart attack.

This "clogged pipe" scenario can occur, but we now know that it's not the cause of most heart attacks.

What's Plaque Really Doing Inside the Artery, Then?

It's not surprising that the clogged pipe theory persisted for so long because the imaging tools used to study and observe coronary arteries gave us only part of the story of plaque development. We could easily identify narrowed arteries outlined on a heart catheterization, and those became the focus of our attention. The problem was, we were limited by image resolution.

We could see plaque's effects on overall vessel diameter, but we couldn't see it in various stages of accumulation or how it really affected lumen diameter and vessel architecture over time.

That changed in 1989 with the advent of intravascular ultrasound (IVUS), a miniature imaging tool that can be snaked into heart arteries to provide a view of vessels from the inside out. IVUS showed, from its unique cross-sectional vantage point, that plaque accumulation can progress quite aggressively before it ever starts to narrow an artery. IVUS also demonstrated plaque rupture—and that really changed our understanding of coronary artery disease.

Although blood vessels are sometimes likened to pipes or conduits, they're much more involved structurally because they have several layers of muscle and tissue. Plaque does not accumulate on the innermost layer of the artery wall (the endothelium) the way corrosion does on the inside wall of a water pipe. Rather, it accumulates *underneath* the endothelium.

In its early stages—and this is key—the accumulation progresses outward, away from the vessel lumen. IVUS shows us that a significant amount of outward accumulation can occur *without ever affecting lumen size* or, as a result, blood flow. In this scenario, traditional imaging tools would show a completely normal-looking artery. So you might have significant atherosclerosis, yet cardiac catheterization would significantly underestimate its severity.

Remember: even though plaque can accumulate for some time without narrowing the artery, that doesn't mean the artery is okay for the time being. Any amount of plaque accumulation is a sign of trouble because its development signals the presence of atherosclerosis, a disease that progresses at different rates in arteries throughout the entire body. And the absence of narrowing doesn't mean a reduced heart attack risk because the plaque in that artery may very well be "unstable," or prone to rupture.

Suppose traditional imaging of your heart showed narrowing in two coronary arteries; one of those appeared to be about 90 percent narrowed and the other about 40 percent. Intuitively,

Additional Info

This is a beautiful example illustrating the necessity for well-designed research. Intuition alone would suggest more severe blockages are more closely linked to future heart attacks. In fact, the opposite is true and led to the pursuit of the actual mechanism: fissuring and rupturing of unstable soft plaques. IVUS made an additional interesting initial discovery. A patient who experiences a ruptured plaque demonstrates an increased likelihood of having a simultaneous second or even third ruptured plaque in a different location. There seems to be a local "environmental" predilection existing within the coronary arterial system that explains this heightened propensity. It is yet to be fully elucidated.

you might conclude that the artery exhibiting 90 percent blockage is the one to worry about. But this isn't the case.

Larger plaques are less prone to rupture, and smaller ones cause most heart attacks. Arteries exhibiting 40 to 50 percent narrowing or even less are more likely to cause heart attacks. The current belief is that these arteries contain "soft" plaque, which makes them unstable and susceptible to abrupt rupture and blockage, known as acute occlusion. This means they're much more dangerous than arteries that show significantly greater narrowing (and that contain mostly hard plaque).

The "Cap" Is Key. Plaque is a biological house of horrors, a collection of biochemical characters—dead tissue, fats, inflammatory blood cells, scar tissue—whose presence in a single location doesn't serve the artery well, particularly when it comes in direct contact with the blood supply. Holding the whole mess in place, so to speak, is a fibrous cap, which is basically scar tissue made of collagen. The fibrous cap is like the burlap tarp covering the compost pile.

Biological interactions inside the plaque can weaken the fibrous cap. In the same way a blemish that develops on the face can bulge and erupt through the skin, plaque contents can weaken the fibrous cap, causing a crack that exposes its internal components. The body treats this event as an injury.

If you accidentally prick one of your fingers with a pin, the blood-clotting response kicks into action, quickly sending blood-clotting components to the site to plug the "leak." When a plaque ruptures, a similar response takes place. The plaque contents are exposed to the bloodstream, particularly the blood-clotting components—platelets, for example—which attach to the fatty accumulations the way chewing gum baking on a hot sidewalk sticks to your shoe.

The platelets launch the blood-clotting process, a normal, protective response to tissue injury, and as the clotting components congregate at the rupture site, the mound, or thrombus, grows in size. But in the confines of an already narrowed artery lumen, the clot is anything but protective.

Although not all plaques are unstable, those that are can be ruinous to heart health. An unstable plaque can transform a 40 to 50 percent narrowing into a 100 percent obstruction in a matter of minutes. So, what was once a virtually harmless, symptomless narrowing is now a life-altering or even life-ending situation. Interestingly, unstable plaque—more often than not—does not critically affect lumen size. So the failure of imaging tools to detect advanced artery narrowing does not mean that your arteries are plaque free.

Plaque Rupture Scenarios. In the aftermath of plaque rupture, several things can happen. Sometimes clotting occurs, but the thrombus formed by the repair isn't large enough to significantly impede blood flow. In fact, this scenario could occur several times before it ever caused symptoms. Think of a series of mild volcanic events long before a cataclysmic eruption.

Another possibility is that the thrombus formed over the plaque disrupts blood flow just enough to cause symptoms such as chest discomfort. And, depending on the individual, that chest pain may or may not be the catalyst for a medical visit.

A third possibility is that the thrombus significantly impedes blood flow and causes heart damage in the form of a heart attack.

Now, having said all this, here's the catch: the presence of coronary artery disease doesn't guarantee that a heart attack is in your future. But, given the risks associated with the presence of atherosclerosis, patients should be very cautious.

Cardiologists are developing methods to identify which patients are at the greatest risk of heart attack from rupture of unstable plaque. And one of their goals, using medical treatments like cholesterol-lowering and antihypertensive medications and lifestyle modification, is to transform unstable plaque into stable plaque to help reduce heart attack risk.

The most common form of heart attack involves unstable plaque resulting in 100 percent obstruction. In a few cases, gradual obstruction develops to near-complete blockage.

During periods of high cardiac stress—such as strong emotion, debilitating illness, or physical exertion—the oxygen supply needed by the heart is quite high. So significant narrowing can interrupt blood flow, which results in heart attack. We see this when hospitalized patients develop "cardiac stressors" while they're awaiting, undergoing, or recovering from noncardiac surgery. Changes in blood pressure and simultaneous blood loss during surgery are two cardiac stressors that develop because oxygen supply is low and the heart's demand for oxygen is high. This can cause heart attack in the hospitalized setting. After noncardiac surgery, a heightened tendency for blood clotting exists. This is termed a prothrombotic state for which the exact mechanism of development is unknown.

• • • *Fast Fact* • • •

Many heart attacks occur in the early morning hours just before or upon awakening. Many hypotheses exist for this occurrence, but the exact reason is yet to be identified. It is felt to be related to a heightened blood-clotting tendency found at that time of day.

• • •

Does the Heart Have Any Protection Against Coronary Artery Disease?

As far as we know, the heart has no internal defense mechanism to protect itself from coronary artery disease. But there's a system in place that helps minimize the risk of tissue damage from artery narrowing. The system consists of vascular channels called collaterals. These are fully functional though comparatively smaller arteries that connect the heart's large arteries. In a healthy heart, the collaterals remain basically unused and "closed."

Think of collaterals this way: you may take the same route to work every day, but along the way, you pass plenty of roads that could serve as alternate routes should your regular route become obstructed by an accident or road work. You wouldn't take those routes unless you were forced to.

In the heart, with all major arteries functioning normally, there isn't enough pressure to force a significant amount of blood into the tiny collaterals. It simply rushes by their channel openings using alternative "major routes." But when significant artery narrowing occurs, it's accompanied by increased pressure transmitted to alternative collateral routes that can force the collaterals to open up. In a sense, they are recruited for duty. That rerouting of the blood supply, in turn, helps direct oxygenated blood to heart tissue that is at risk of undernourishment because of narrowing. Collateral circulation, then, is a built-in protective measure against a reduction in blood supply.

The system can be so effective that even in the presence of a significantly narrowed artery, patients experience no symptoms and no tissue damage. For someone with coronary artery disease, development of an extensive collateral network can be a good

Did You Know?

A 100 percent coronary artery blockage accompanied by extensive collateral blood vessels does not necessarily result in heart damage. This is because the narrowing developed slowly, permitting collateral vessel recruitment and utilization. Look at it this way—collaterals are an internal defense mechanism to guard against heart damage and are a very good thing.

thing. It helps prevent heart muscle damage caused by heart attack. However, a working collateral network can also mask coronary artery disease.

Heart Attack Symptoms

About 30 to 40 percent of patients who suffer from a heart attack, particularly women and diabetic patients, experience no symptoms at all. Should symptoms be present, these patients tend not to exhibit classic heart attack symptoms: crushing chest discomfort that streaks up around the neck or down through the arm. Less typical symptoms may include a sensation of indigestion or mid-back discomfort between the shoulder blades.

Regardless of whether symptoms are experienced by men or women, sometimes they are dismissed, and the possibility of a heart attack is never considered. This underscores the importance of patient education—and also of exercise.

Exercise can help you stay attuned to signals your body is sending. For instance, most people who exercise regularly are aware of their exercise capacity. Most of us plateau at some point, and that's okay. But if over time you find that you're regressing from that plateau, and it can't be attributed to hot weather, fatigue, illness, or stress, there could a problem. If your exercise capacity starts diminishing and you develop symptoms you've never before experienced, such as chest discomfort and shortness of breath, see your physician.

The most common symptoms of advancing coronary artery disease or potential heart attack are shortness of breath and chest discomfort, particularly during physical exertion. Fainting and fatigue are also possible. Education will help ensure that such symptoms, rather than a heart attack, spur a visit to a physician. And, for those who are sedentary with undiagnosed, developing atherosclerosis, exercise may precipitate symptoms earlier and trigger that visit to a physician.

Heart Attack Symptoms in Women

The most common heart attack symptoms experienced by women are:

- Pain or discomfort in the center of the chest
- Pain or discomfort in areas of the upper body, such as the arms, back, jaw, neck, or stomach
- Shortness of breath, cold sweat, nausea, fatigue, or lightheadedness.

Although these are similar to men's symptoms, the wrinkle here is that women are also likely to experience atypical symptoms without chest discomfort, such as nausea and vomiting, back or jaw pain, and shortness of breath. Some women may have no noticeable symptoms at all.

Another concern is the lack of awareness of the extent of heart disease in women. As we noted in chapter 1, women who report symptoms or believe that they have heart problems may not be taken as seriously as men by family members or healthcare providers, even when they're in an emergency department.

So, for the women reading this book: be your own advocates. If you think there's something wrong with your heart, trust your instincts. If you feel you're not getting proper attention from your healthcare provider, either be more persistent or find a provider who will take your concerns seriously. Pay attention to your risk factors and work with your physician to manage your smoking, cholesterol, weight, blood pressure, or diabetes. And be mindful of new symptoms that may signal a cardiac problem.

In terms of chest discomfort, most health and medical sources use the term *chest pain,* but *discomfort* is more accurate. If you ask a patient who is experiencing a coronary artery event, "Are you experiencing pain?" the answer may be "No." If you ask the same patient, "Are you experiencing discomfort in or around your chest?"

the answer may well by "Yes." Discomfort is a better descriptor to use because it can encompass both pain and pressure symptoms. Remember also that pain perception is subjective. Pain to one person may be pressure to another. A "light" discomfort to one may be a "severe" discomfort to another. That's why it is so important to remain attuned to your body and the differing signals it may be sending your way. It is also why I am such a big advocate of regular exercise. I am a firm believer that regular aerobic exercise not only helps prevent chronic disease, including heart disease, but it also gives you the ability to gauge any new symptoms with greater precision using your baseline exercise capacity as a barometer.

Presumption about the heart's location in the chest can also cause confusion about symptoms. Many people think that the heart resides on the left side of the chest. In fact, it resides directly underneath the breast bone (the sternum), in the center of the chest, and it is slightly tilted to the left. So the cardiac apex, which is the lowermost anatomical point of the heart (the tip of the heart), is situated slightly to the left.

But heart attack-induced pain is not always left-sided. It's often what we call substernal (in the middle of the chest). Rather than causing a specific point of discomfort, the pain is diffuse within a particular region of the chest, larger than a dime or quarter and often depicted as the size of one's clenched fist. Inhaling or exhaling deeply typically won't affect the discomfort.

The discomfort often radiates to the throat, neck, jaw, teeth, shoulders, and arms. It's often on the inside of the left arm that we typically feel an aching discomfort that radiates down to the elbow and sometimes to the hand. Occasionally the pain will occur in both arms. For some people, the only symptom experienced will be arm discomfort. Regardless of the site of that discomfort, people typically can't find a position that relieves the pain. Nor do they find relief by ingesting liquids, popping antacids, or taking deep breaths.

When heart discomfort or pain does develop, it's unrelenting, although typically only for several minutes (not seconds or

Worry or Not to Worry?

A completely normal, healthy body can develop all sorts of fleeting aches and pains that aren't heart related. It's the symptoms that linger for minutes that you should worry about. Most of the time, they *will* get your attention.

The following symptoms are unlikely to signal a heart attack:

- Momentary chest discomfort, often characterized as a lightning bolt or electrical shock
- Pinpoint chest discomfort that worsens with positional changes or during breathing
- Chest discomfort that seems to get better with exercise

hours), and then it subsides if it is a temporary interruption of blood flow. In the presence of a sustained coronary artery blockage, a heart attack transpires. In this situation, the discomfort is ongoing, often occurring alongside shortness of breath, sweating, nausea, profound fatigue, and a sense of unease, anxiety, or of feeling ill. Many patients exhibit the Levine sign, a classic heart attack clue, whereby a person holds a clenched fist on top of the chest to draw a physician's attention to the source and sensation of the pain (the clenched fist equals tightness or pressure).

In general, heart attack symptoms last longer than a few minutes and up to a range of 30 to 120 minutes. Despite the above description, symptom severity can vary greatly.

How Do I Know When I'm Experiencing Symptoms of a Heart Attack?

If you feel that you are experiencing heart attack symptoms, it's better to err on the side of caution and visit a physician or emergency department. The symptoms below can mimic a heart attack, but when in doubt, please check it out:

- Pulmonary emboli (blood clots that travel to the lungs) cause severe chest discomfort that mimics a heart attack. This is a medical emergency.

- Aortic dissection, a tear in the aorta, occurs most often in people with high blood pressure. Its symptoms are similar to those of heart attack. Seek emergency treatment.

- Chest discomfort that gets worse with eating (postprandial angina) can signal a problem in the heart or a gastrointestinal problem. If such episodes occur regularly, see your doctor.

- Esophageal spasm (irregular contractions of the muscles in the "tube" through which we swallow food) can cause chest discomfort similar to angina, complicating the diagnosis of heart attack.

- Cholecystitis, inflammation of the gallbladder, can cause chest discomfort.

- Hiatal hernia (a condition in which a portion of the stomach protrudes upward into the chest cavity through an opening in the diaphragm) can cause chest discomfort.

What Is Angina?

Angina, or angina pectoris, is a classic heart disease symptom. It signals the vessel narrowing caused by advanced coronary artery disease. Angina is the heart's way of telling you that some part of it isn't getting enough blood. Angina commonly arises when a coronary artery lumen is significantly narrowed, anywhere from 70 to 100 percent.

Angina doesn't arise in all individuals with heart disease, but when it does, it can cause significant discomfort or pain in and around the chest. This is sometimes called an angina attack.

Angina can be grouped into several categories:

- **Stable angina,** the most common type, is predictable, occurs in a regular pattern, and fades after a few minutes with rest and medication. It's also a signal that heart disease is present and there's an increased risk of heart attack.

- **Unstable angina** is a highly lethal condition and heralds an impending heart attack. It doesn't act like a lightning bolt; rather, it can begin, last a few minutes, may or may not disappear when you rest, and then resurface when you resume physical activity. Unlike stable angina, its onset is unpredictable. Unstable angina is considered a medical emergency and means that it's time to get to a hospital for evaluation.

- **Continuous angina** indicates that a heart attack has likely just occurred. However, even during a heart attack, angina may come and go. Blood flow is fleetingly restored as the body's own system for degrading clots attempts to open a clogged artery, a process called spontaneous thrombolysis.

How Do Doctors Confirm Heart Attacks?

An electrocardiogram measures the heart's electrical activity and produces a paper "strip" that exhibits telltale patterns of normal and abnormal heart activity. One pattern is called an "ST-segment elevation MI" (myocardial infarct) and is the telltale sign of a sudden, 100 percent obstruction of the coronary artery. In fact, the ST-segment elevation MI is the classic finding of an acute heart attack. It's as if someone tied a stitch around the coronary artery tight enough to completely cut off blood flow through the vessel.

An echocardiogram measures ejection fraction. Ejection fraction is the percentage of blood ejected from the left ventricle with each heart contraction. Under normal circumstances, roughly two-thirds of the blood in the left ventricle is ejected during contraction. But during a heart attack, depending upon the extent of damage, the ejection fraction falls below normal.

• • • *Fast Fact* • • •

An electrocardiogram, when abnormal in the setting of anginal chest pain, provides valuable additive information including localizing what coronary artery is obstructed and permitting an estimate of the size of the ongoing heart muscle damage. Even in the presence of a heart attack, the electrocardiogram can be normal or demonstrate at most a slight deviation from normal. In this circumstance, additional testing is essential.

• • •

Measuring ejection fraction during and following a heart attack is important to assess the damage to the heart's pumping function. The ejection fraction range also dictates which medications are selected and how doses are administered. Ejection fraction is closely correlated with prognosis: the lower the ejection fraction, the worse the outcome. In small heart attacks, the ejection fraction is minimally affected and is generally above 50 percent. In a moderate heart attack, the ejection fraction may be in the 40 percent range. In a large heart attack or after two moderate heart attacks, the ejection fraction falls into the 20 to 25 percent range or even lower. The echocardiogram can also localize the area of heart damage and together with the electrocardiogram predict with good accuracy which coronary artery is responsible for the heart damage. The echocardiogram provides additional valuable information including an assessment of the heart valves and pressures within the heart, both pieces of data having a significant impact on patient treatment recommendations.

Do Heart Attacks Leave Scars?

Any assault on the body's tissue can result in scarring, and it's no different with heart attack. Heart attacks result in scars on the heart best characterized as irreversible damage to heart muscle.

Heart muscle is similar to any other muscle, in the sense that it has contractile properties. With each electrical pulse generated from the heart's pacemaker, the cells respond by creating a uniform wave of contraction, which results in the pumping action that maintains constant blood circulation throughout the body. To ensure that this process occurs efficiently and effectively, the heart muscle needs to remain healthy.

In patients who have a "small" heart attack, a comparatively small amount of heart tissue sustains damage, leaving the heart with a fairly good pumping capacity. The individual is able to maintain a quality of life without significant functional limitations. In other words, engaging in rigorous physical activity poses no problem.

Heart attacks that cause a medium or large scar on the heart can significantly impair the heart's pumping function and its ability to maintain adequate cardiac output for delivering blood and oxygen to the body.

Even with a medium or large area of tissue scarring, the heart can respond to demands to circulate blood, and heart attack survivors may experience no symptoms when the body is relaxed or at rest. However, things can change significantly if the heart is asked to do more during periods of physical exertion. When oxygen demand from the peripheral tissues increases significantly, the heart must respond in kind with greater cardiac output. But significant tissue damage prevents an adequate response. Therefore, performing everyday activities, such as walking up a flight of stairs, walking long distances, or carrying a bag of groceries, may be a struggle.

People who are sedentary and experience significant tissue damage from a heart attack may develop complications such as shortness of breath even when they're resting. This combination

Fibrosis: The Heart Attack Scar

When heart tissue dies, it's transformed into fibrotic tissue, characterized by an infiltration of smooth muscle cells and cells called fibroblasts. This scar tissue develops the same way you might develop a permanent scar on your skin after trauma from a deep cut or wound. In the case of the heart—and this is important—the fibrotic tissue has no contractile ability. Therefore, it has no active pumping function and instead merely takes up space in the heart.

of symptoms is a sign of congestive heart failure, a condition in which the heart can't maintain an adequate cardiac output. Pressure builds in the lungs, causing shortness of breath, as well as fluid retention in the lungs and peripheral tissues.

What Should I Do if I Think I Have Symptoms of a Heart Attack?

When warning symptoms of coronary insufficiency or acute heart attack develop, getting to a hospital immediately is extremely important, because clot-dissolving medications—thrombolytics—can be administered to open clogged blood vessels. These agents are effective in restoring adequate blood flow in the coronary arteries of up to 80 percent of patients who receive them.

Assuming a person gets to a hospital shortly after heart attack symptoms arise, heart management is dictated by the cardiac resources of the medical center handling the case. If you're taken to a center that has an active interventional cardiology program and a catheterization lab on the premises, it's likely that you'll undergo cardiac catheterization that includes angioplasty and stenting in lieu of clot-dissolving medications. This is accomplished by snaking a slender tool—a balloon-tipped catheter—to the site of vessel narrowing (occlusion). There, the balloon is inflated to widen the artery, and the stent is deployed to maintain the widening achieved by balloon angioplasty. (For more about this procedure, see chapter 8.)

Remember, a reduction or complete loss of blood supply due to a clogged coronary artery poses a significant threat to the portion of the heart that relies on that vessel for oxygenated blood. Starved of blood, cardiac cells—the fundamental units of heart muscle—begin dying off within minutes. So the longer it takes to get blood flow restored, the greater the extent of tissue damage. In other words, time is muscle.

This doesn't mean that if hospitalization doesn't occur within minutes of the heart attack, you will die or that significant tissue scarring is inevitable. Keep in mind that major arteries go through a number of branchings and that these branches subdivide within the heart tissue. This, along with collateral blood vessels, helps ensure an adequate supply of blood to the tissues in the event that the blood supply is partially and temporarily cut off, as in a heart attack.

Studies have shown that there's an approximate six-hour window for interventions such as administering clot-dissolving medications, angioplasty, and stenting. In some patients whose persistent chest discomfort and electrocardiogram abnormalities continue, interventions up to twelve hours have been demonstrated to be

Additional Info

It's also a good idea to chew at least one 325 mg aspirin should you suspect a heart attack. Aspirin possesses an antiplatelet effect, diminishing the stickiness of the circulating clot forming blood cells called platelets.

helpful. Individualization of the patient's care is the key. Swift intervention can keep the area of infarct—tissue irreversibly damaged by the heart attack—as small as possible by maintaining sufficient pumping capacity.

Certainly, by six hours, groups of cells have sustained irreversible damage. But there's a gradation of damage—almost a series of concentric zones, with the innermost zone (the tissue most dependent upon blood from the obstructed vessel) being the most damaged and the surrounding zones (which also draw blood from other major coronary vessels or branches) less damaged. This means that hours after a heart attack, there's a zone or rim of living tissue still vulnerable to further damage. If intervention restores blood flow, the risk to this zone is reduced. The point is that prompt intervention can limit the area of infarct and prevent further complications, such as remodeling (enlarging) of the heart and aneurysm (abnormal ballooning) at the infarct site due to the dead tissue's weakened state.

It Can't Happen to Me

Denial is a common theme among people who have heart attack symptoms. But that denial must be overcome by learning heart attack symptoms and listening intently to our own bodies. Heart disease *is* the leading cause of death in the United States, and it strikes indiscriminately across lines of gender, age, and ethnicity.

Jim's Story

It was Friday evening, rush hour, Christmas Eve, 1999. Jim, 47, was twenty minutes from his home, wife, and three children. Like most of his fellow commuters, his mind was racing, thinking about the holiday, the gifts still to be wrapped, the visits with family and friends, the precious time away from work. The steady, daily supply of coffee, Coke, and cigarettes no doubt contributed to his hyperanxiety, but it had been a stressful few weeks at work, and now, as he steered his car toward home—and refuge—the stress began to manifest itself in his shoulders. Jim tried massaging them to shake the tension, to restore some semblance of calm. It didn't work. Instead, the tightness migrated to his chest. He tried to preoccupy himself with his Christmas to-do list and to avoid thinking about his work at the local hospital, where a pile of credentialing cases sat on his desk. That pile seemed to be growing exponentially, waiting to be processed so that 100 physicians could practice in compliance with the law. What perfect timing. Christmas Eve. There was no end to it, and the work could never get finished fast enough.

The tightness in his chest persisted; then he felt something odd going on with his breathing. He was having trouble expanding his chest to get enough air into his lungs. Instinctively—although illogically—he pulled a cigarette from the ever-present pack in his shirt pocket and lit up. Smoking always calmed him, and he needed that nicotine solace now. Oddly, inhaling a menthol light on this day, at this moment, didn't help. In fact, he was feeling progressively worse. He added nausea to the growing list of annoyances plaguing him on this now interminable drive home. What was going on?

He'd been a pack-and-a-half per day smoker since age 16. He had relatives—his mother's side of the family—who had dropped over dead from heart attacks. His diet would make a cardiologist squirm (and reach for the nearest supply of statins). But none of these facts, these red flags, occurred to him now. All he knew was that something wasn't right, that he wanted to be home, and that he wanted it all to stop.

The tightness in his shoulders, the inability to catch his breath or fill his lungs with air, the odd sensation in his chest—all of it persisted. Then, out of nowhere, he broke into a cold sweat. Not just on his hands, forehead, and underarms, but all over his body. He was drenched almost from head to toe, and it all happened in seconds. He began sensing, grudgingly, that something was wrong medically, but he still wasn't putting the pieces together. In fact, if someone had asked him before he got in the car that evening to name even one heart disease symptom, he would have drawn a blank.

He focused on getting to his house. Finally, he was on his street, with the driveway and garage in sight. He parked the car and made his way inside through the kitchen, dropping his briefcase in stride. He trudged determinedly by his wife, barely saying hello, and climbed the stairs to his bedroom to lie down.

Lying on his bed, he really began to get scared. The tightness in his shoulders and chest was conspicuously painful, and he struggled with each breath. He was terrified but too scared to get back up. He wanted to call for his wife, but he could barely talk, much less yell, and it seemed to take forever to get her attention. She finally came upstairs and into the bedroom, somewhat reluctantly, because she never expected that her husband would be crying out to her for help. This was a man who was never sick, who hiked challenging mountain slopes, who trained for the hikes by donning bulky hiking shoes and a backpack full of weights. He was in excellent physical shape; if he was overweight, it was by ounces, not pounds. But she looked at him and saw a tense, pale, sweaty, and desperate stranger. "Karen. Call 911. Call 911 now," Jim said, in frantic exhaustion.

During the interim, Jim's 12-year-old daughter Theresa trod carefully into the bedroom. She knew something was wrong; she was scared but didn't say much. Instead, she got onto the bed, put her arms around her father, and hugged him hard. Suddenly, just for a few moments, Jim felt relief from the chest pain, and he hugged her back. It was the first time since the symptoms started that he had felt any relief.

The paramedics arrived in minutes—just the sight of them was a relief. They asked several direct questions, took multiple blood-pressure measurements and pulse readings, and then gave Jim two small nitroglycerin tablets, which he dissolved by putting under his tongue.

"Do you think you can walk out of here?" one asked.

Jim was feeling less frantic now. "Yes," he answered.

The paramedics helped him out of bed and escorted him downstairs. On the way out of the bedroom, Jim snatched his cigarettes and lighter from the dresser top, then spent the better part of the chaperoned journey down the stairway trying to put these trusted accessories into the breast pocket of his button-down work shirt. Then it occurred to him: he had no pocket, because he'd taken his shirt off before falling into bed. Now he was wearing only a T-shirt, and it clearly had no pockets. The futility of the act, the pain, the labored breathing, the realization that he was heading to the hospital for emergency medical care, and the pack of menthol lights in his palm—suddenly the facts converged and in an instant, he took a last look at the cigarettes and lighter, and defiantly tossed both over his shoulder. It would be the last time he held a pack of cigarettes in his hands.

Once at the local hospital, things moved quickly, with the emergency team wasting no time getting x-rays, performing an electrocardiogram, pushing fluids intravenously, and drawing blood for enzyme testing. Initial results revealed a blockage that, while significant, appeared to be in a place where it caused minimal tissue damage. Almost immediately, the team began administering the clot-dissolving drug streptokinase. Then, every ten seconds or so, someone would ask Jim about the pain level in his chest. When he arrived at the hospital, he rated it a seven or eight out of ten; as the night progressed, he kept downgrading it. The streptokinase was working, helping to gradually break down the clot so that blood could flow more freely through his plaque-laden vessel. By bedtime, he was rating the pain a one. There was some residual tightness, but he felt much better. He was tucked away in a bed by 9 P.M., Christmas Eve.

The two cardiologists who performed the catheterization laid out the situation for Jim on Monday, two days after Christmas. Their presentation was brief and matter-of-fact: "You've got major blockages throughout your heart. You need open-heart surgery. We're proposing five grafts, using vessels taken from inside your chest and leg. We want to do this ASAP." There was no mention of managing the situation with medical therapy or stents or some combination thereof. "You need open-heart surgery—now."

During that face-the-music meeting, the cardiologists asked Jim whether anyone else in his family had ever had heart problems. It was then that Jim realized he had unintentionally repressed a family history of heart disease. It turns out that, in addition to heart disease, smoking and caffeine addiction ran in the family.

Jim has three brothers—two older, one younger—and all are doing well. The two older brothers had smoked but quit; the younger brother is trying to quit. A cousin on his mother's side of the family, who was overweight, a heavy smoker, and a coffee lover, died in his early 40s from a massive heart attack. An autopsy showed pervasive atherosclerosis throughout the arteries. Jim's father had had a heart attack in his 50s but thankfully survived. He was able to manage the condition with medicine. Jim was in his mid-20s at the time. His mother's sister, who was hooked on coffee, Coke, and cigarettes, died at age 50 from a massive heart attack. Her heart resembled the cousin's.

Aftermath

The surgery, which lasted six hours, went off without a hitch. His medical team got Jim up and walking within twenty-four hours.

He began his recuperation by doing laps around the floor of the ward, IV in tow, increasing the distance each day of the five he was hospitalized postoperatively. Immediately after, he started on aspirin, which helps prevent strokes and heart attacks; a beta-blocker; an ACE inhibitor (a medication that dilates blood vessels, reduces blood pressure and therefore reduces the workload on the heart); and a statin.

After being discharged from the hospital, he joined the cardiac rehabilitation program for three sessions a week. For the ten weeks that he was away from his job, he worked out on treadmills, stationary cycles, and stair climbers. There was constant monitoring of blood pressure and heart rate, and a steady supply of pulse-rate targets to try to reach. The objective was to rebuild stamina and lung capacity. During the weeks in cardiac rehab, he learned how to exercise safely, using warm-ups before exercise (and intervals of rest during) to prevent overexertion.

One significant challenge immediately after surgery involved breathing. After surgery, Jim felt as if he had significantly less room inside his chest. He couldn't expand it, couldn't take a deep breath, couldn't fill his lungs as he was used to doing. There were a lot of shallow breaths for many months. This was the longest part of the recuperation for Jim, who was used to being physically active. He couldn't run for a very long time; he couldn't jog. He could only walk.

Eventually, Jim fell in love with walking, and it remains the key component of his exercise regimen. Three or four days a week, weather permitting, he tries to get out of the office for a brisk forty-five-minute walk. Cigarettes and caffeine are addictions of the past, as are fast-food joints. In fact, he's had to recalibrate his budget to accommodate eating at restaurants where patrons order from menus. Although he characterizes the heart-healthy diet he had while hospitalized as tasteless, his diet outside of the hospital is anything but and consists primarily of salads and lightly grilled poultry, fish, or lean beef. Today, he's less stressed out at work, his health is stable, and he's happy to be alive, pursuing a renewed love of music and planning future hikes and camping trips with his wife and kids.

In the weeks and months after his open-heart surgery, as Jim learned more about the procedure and its risks and challenges, he reflected on that conversation with the cardiologists. "They really didn't tell me anything about what to expect, how the procedure would be done, what the risks were. And I don't know if that is good or bad. If they had given me too much info, maybe I would have gotten anxious and backed out." On the other hand, if he wanted to get well—and he did—there were no other options. His heart needed help. And Jim was all for getting better. He had no desire to live his life with a time bomb in his chest. "I said, 'Whatever you want to do, I'm all yours.' I didn't want to walk out of the hospital at high risk for another attack because maybe next time I won't be so lucky about making it to the hospital in time."

Can I Fully Recover from a Heart Attack?

In a basic way, your level of heart function after a heart attack determines your prognosis. If you have remaining normal heart function in the wake of a heart attack and then undergo an intervention such as bypass surgery, your prognosis is very good. But if a heart attack causes severe heart dysfunction, and that dysfunction persists even after surgical intervention, you're more apt to develop arrhythmias, congestive heart failure, or sudden cardiac death.

The greater the amount of heart muscle affected, the greater the likelihood of problems such as heart remodeling, aneurysm formation, valve leakage, and so on. So the size of the infarct dictates how susceptible you will be to one of the conditions outlined below.

Arrhythmias. Arrhythmias are heart rhythm disorders common among people who have coronary artery disease or have had heart attacks. The problems arise as the result of inadequate blood supply to heart tissue.

There are basically two types of heart arrhythmias: those that originate from the heart's upper chambers (the atria), called atrial arrhythmias, and those that originate from lower chambers (the ventricles), called ventricular arrhythmias. Atrial arrhythmias are typically less dangerous than ventricular arrhythmias.

The most common atrial arrhythmia is atrial fibrillation, in which the atria incessantly beat in a discordant and chaotic fashion, between 400 and 600 times per minute. Fortunately, the atrioventricular or AV node, the heart's backup pacemaker, also serves as a filter or gatekeeper, preventing transmission of the bulk of those unwanted signals from the atria. (By contrast, ventricular contractions at that rate would quickly result in death.)

Under normal circumstances and in the absence of cardiac medications, just 20 to 25 percent of the abnormal 400 to 600 atrial beats per minute are transmitted to the ventricles. So in addition to helping ensure propagation of electrical signals through cardiac tissue, the AV node serves as a gatekeeper against unwanted signals to protect the heart. Electrical impulses that otherwise would get past the AV node can be managed with medications that also help control heart rate.

Atrial flutter is another common atrial arrhythmia. It's a bit less chaotic than atrial fibrillation and is caused by an abnormal electrical circuit (also called a reentrant arrhythmia), typically located within the right atrium. Atrial flutter results in approximately 300 atrial contractions per minute. Again, the AV node serves as a protector of the ventricles, allowing the transmission of only 20 to 25 percent of the errant signals.

Atrial arrhythmias are best treated with medication; however, if such treatment proves ineffective or if the drugs' side effects become problematic, some patients may be advised to undergo radiofrequency ablation. In this procedure, a catheter with an electrode at its tip is used to deliver a small dose of radiofrequency energy to destroy a small number of heart electrical fibers responsible for conducting the extra electrical impulses causing the rhythm disturbance.

Atrial fibrillation and atrial flutter can cause heart palpitations, lightheadedness, weakness, near-fainting, low blood pressure, sweating, nausea, and angina in some cases. Less commonly, atrial fibrillation can lead to heart attack or congestive heart failure, particularly during periods of sustained rapid heart rates.

More worrisome are ventricular arrhythmias, as they can cause loss of consciousness and sudden cardiac death, which is due to the heart's inability to pump blood. Ventricular arrhythmias are often associated with interrupted blood flow to the heart or scarring caused by heart attack; both can cause tissue dysfunction that results in electrical irritability and, in turn, ventricular arrhythmia.

The most common ventricular arrhythmia is ventricular tachycardia, a regular but abnormally fast contraction rate (150 to 225 beats per minute) emanating from the lower pumping chambers. This condition severely compromises pumping efficiency. Very little blood actually leaves the ventricles, and cardiac output is significantly hampered.

The situation can worsen as the body's tissues send signals for more blood, and the ventricles respond by contracting even faster—to the point that they begin to quiver, a condition called ventricular fibrillation. At this point, virtually no blood leaves the ventricles. Without immediate intervention such as cardiopulmonary resuscitation, ventricular fibrillation is lethal.

Again, scar tissue from a heart attack is the culprit. The interface between fibrotic (nonfunctioning cardiac tissue) and normal cardiac muscle can precipitate problems in the electrical circuitry of the heart—so-called reentrant arrhythmias.

Ventricular arrhythmias can be managed with heart rhythm medications that help control abnormal ventricular electrical activity. Or patients might be advised to undergo surgery for a life-saving implantable cardioverter-defibrillator (ICD), a small device that monitors the heart for irregular ventricular activity. These devices emit electrical signals that terminate a ventricular arrhythmia and can "shock" the heart, if need be, to restore normal rhythm during

Did You Know?

There are specific criteria for ICD implantation developed in response to findings from carefully designed large-scale research projects involving thousands of patients. In general, the lower the ejection fraction after a heart attack, the greater the propensity for a serious ventricular arrhythmia arising. An ejection fraction after a heart attack of 35 percent or less is generally the value utilized to decide if an ICD should be implanted.

episodes of persistent ventricular rhythm disturbance. If ventricular fibrillation persists, it causes loss of consciousness within seconds. The ICD in essence can be a lifesaver.

Heart Failure. One of the most costly, debilitating, and lethal legacies of heart attack is congestive heart failure, a chronic condition in which the heart gradually loses its pumping effectiveness. Heart failure is incredibly challenging to treat because it has many forms and causes, affects several body systems, and has no cure. The best treatment is to prevent it from occurring in the first place.

In the end stages of heart failure, an available but scarce option for prolonging life is heart transplantation. (Several efforts are underway, however, including those at the Cleveland Clinic, to develop effective transplant alternatives such as artificial hearts.)

Though somewhat cumbersome, implantable devices called left ventricular assist devices (LVADs) can assist the heart in pumping blood. LVADs were developed to manage heart failure patients awaiting transplant and were thought of as temporary therapy. Because suitable hearts for transplantation are in short supply, cardiologists are also using LVADs for "destination" therapy, meaning that the device is permanently implanted in lieu of transplantation.

It's not a perfect solution and comes with complications, including infection and blood clotting in internal tubing.

The hallmark of congestive heart failure is fluid congestion: abnormal blood pooling that accumulates in the veins, arteries, lungs, and other organs, as well as the heart chambers themselves, due to lost pumping capacity. Fluid accumulation, also called edema, can be especially noticeable in the legs, which typically swell. Edema also can enlarge the liver.

Congestive heart failure can develop after heart attack in one of several ways:

- A heart attack can cause great tissue damage, significantly increasing the pumping burden on the nonaffected muscle.

- The recurrent arrhythmias (atrial or ventricular) that develop in the aftermath of heart attack can fatigue the heart muscle with recurrent, rapid beating.

- A heart attack occurs in a person who has, or develops, valvular disease.

One thing is certain: heart failure is never a good prognosis, particularly when accompanied by coronary artery disease.

One problem associated with heart failure is elevated pressure inside the heart, particularly inside the left ventricle. An increase in pressure there, called elevated left ventricular end diastolic pressure, impairs the left ventricle's ability to properly fill with blood. Blood therefore stagnates within the left atrium, the chamber above the left ventricle. Over time, the pooling of blood in the upper chamber stretches the atrial walls, enlarging the chamber and setting the stage for rhythm problems, such as atrial fibrillation or atrial flutter.

The pressure increase also gets transmitted backward, virtually along the same path the blood takes to reach the heart—moving from the heart's left chambers, through the lungs and pulmonary blood vessels, to the heart's right chambers, and back to the abdominal organs, liver, and lower extremities. That's what causes swelling in the belly and legs—all the cardiovascular pressures are elevated in reverse, impeding the return of blood to the heart from the peripheral circulation. (Within the lungs, this increased pressure causes shortness of breath and poor exercise intolerance.)

Once heart failure develops, there's no turning back; symptoms must be managed with medications. Also, patients can develop life-threatening decompensated heart failure, which includes low blood pressure and excessive lung fluid, or pulmonary edema, that hinders oxygen transfer.

Heart attack can also kill muscle cells in one of the two papillary muscles that form the supporting apparatus for the mitral valve. The mitral valve separates the heart's left atrium from its left ventricle. Scarring of the papillary muscles shortens and stiffens the valve, impairing proper closure. The result is mitral valve leakage.

A large heart attack that affects a significant portion of heart tissue will enlarge the left ventricle over time. This in turn distorts the natural shape of the mitral valve annulus, the supporting structure on which the mitral valve sits. Such distortion prevents the mitral valve leaflets from closing properly and also results in leakage.

Red Flag

Mitral regurgitation in the presence of weakened heart muscle is not a good sign. It can substantially contribute to the development and persistence of congestive heart failure. Medications help but do not cure the valve leak. Instead, the aim of medication administration is to reduce the pressures within the heart. This works with variable success. In cases of advanced mitral valve leakage and refractory congestive heart failure symptoms, open heart surgery in the form of mitral valve repair or replacement is often best.

Heart Attack Begets Heart Attack

Unfortunately, a first heart attack can be followed by a second. This isn't surprising, given that heart attack is a sign of coronary artery disease, and coronary artery disease doesn't magically disappear once a heart attack occurs. Without significant lifestyle changes and management with medications, coronary artery disease will progress.

So if you've had a heart attack and have no desire to repeat the experience, you really need to make significant life changes and work with your physician on managing your weight, blood pressure, and, if you have diabetes, your blood sugar levels. Taking your prescribed medication is critical.

Another important fact: a second heart attack kills more healthy muscle tissue. After two heart attacks, the heart is straining to beat effectively. And with significantly less functional heart tissue to keep things running, the stakes are much higher for developing arrhythmias, aneurysms, valve problems, heart failure, and a shortened life span.

Not surprisingly, treatment gets tougher and more complicated in the wake of a second heart attack. Medications tend to be less effective because of a reduction in viable (living) heart tissue. Several factors dictate the likelihood of a second heart attack:

- The extent of coronary artery disease in heart vessels beyond the one that caused the first heart attack.

- The extent of viable heart muscle tissue in the zones bordering the infarct zone that survived the heart attack. The surviving heart tissue in this area can actually increase the risk of heart attack if an adequate blood supply is not reestablished.

- The success of lifestyle modification efforts and the degree of compliance with prescribed medication.
- The medication types and doses selected.

Can a Heart Attack Be Prevented?

The terms primary and secondary prevention are often used when discussing heart disease management. Primary prevention refers to lifestyle and behavioral changes in the absence of known coronary artery disease: quitting smoking, taking up exercise, cutting back on fat intake. Everything we read about Jim doing after his surgery is what you could be doing right now: these proactive steps can prevent the development of atherosclerosis and minimize the risk of heart attack.

Secondary prevention refers to implementing the lifestyle and behavioral changes described above *after* a diagnosis of coronary artery disease is made—this is what Jim had to do, since for him the heart attack was a near-fatal wake-up call. It also means undergoing interventions such as angioplasty and stenting when needed, and taking cholesterol-lowering drugs after a heart attack has occurred. Secondary prevention is designed to halt further atherosclerosis development, stabilize plaque, and mitigate plaque rupture and to prevent a second heart attack.

Chapter 4

Risk Factors

The main way we gauge the likelihood of heart disease and heart attack is by taking an inventory of risk factors. A risk factor is something that increases the likelihood that you'll develop heart disease or that you'll experience a heart attack. There are two types of risk factors: those that can be affected by lifestyle and behavior changes, called modifiable risk factors; and those that cannot, called nonmodifiable risk factors. You already know some of them, perhaps all of them. And you know from chapter 1 that if there is any one modifiable behavior that poses the greatest danger to the heart, it is smoking. Unfortunately, this is the risk factor that smokers seem to ignore.

The key culprits of modifiable risk factors include smoking, high blood pressure, high cholesterol, diabetes, and obesity. (High cholesterol is explored further in chapter 5.) Of all risk factors, smoking and weight can be the most difficult to manage or modify. Smoking is highly addictive, pleasurable to some, and, for most smokers, a stress management tool. Not surprisingly, many smokers find it difficult to kick the habit. As for being overweight, there's a genetic influence. That means that for some people, weight isn't just a matter of self-control or overindulging. Nevertheless, research has shown that when overweight individuals lose even a small percentage of overall weight, they experience benefits—such as reduced blood pressure and lowered cholesterol levels—that can help protect against heart attack. The mysteries and challenges of nicotine addiction, overweight, and obesity won't be resolved in this book, but readers should understand that they are complex issues. In most cases, these issues are best addressed by heightened self-discipline.

Understanding Risk Factors for Heart Disease

What Are Some Modifiable Risk Factors?

Tobacco Smoke. Smokers' risk of developing coronary heart disease is two to four times that of nonsmokers.[*] Cigarette smoking is a powerful independent risk factor for sudden cardiac death in patients with coronary heart disease; smokers have about twice the risk of nonsmokers. Cigarette smoking also acts with other risk factors to greatly increase the risk for coronary heart disease. People who smoke cigars or pipes seem to have a higher risk of death from coronary heart disease (and possibly stroke), but their risk isn't as great as cigarette smokers'. Exposure to other people's smoke increases the risk of heart disease even for nonsmokers.

High Blood Cholesterol. As blood LDL cholesterol rises, so does risk of coronary heart disease. When other risk factors (like high blood pressure and tobacco smoke) are present, this risk increases even more. A person's cholesterol level is also affected by age, sex, heredity, activity level, and diet.

---

[*] Risk Factors are reproduced with permission of the American Heart Association, *www.americanheart.org* © 2006, American Heart Association.

High Blood Pressure. High blood pressure increases the heart's workload, causing the heart to thicken and become stiffer. It also increases your risk of stroke, heart attack, kidney failure, and congestive heart failure. When high blood pressure exists with obesity, smoking, high blood cholesterol levels, or diabetes the risk of heart attack or stroke increases greatly.

Physical Inactivity. An inactive lifestyle is a risk factor for coronary heart disease. Regular, moderate-to-vigorous physical activity helps prevent heart and blood vessel disease. The more vigorous the activity, the greater your benefits. Yet even moderate-intensity activities help if done regularly and long term. Exercise can help control blood cholesterol, diabetes, and obesity, as well as help lower blood pressure in some people.

Obesity and Overweight. People who have excess body fat—especially if most of it is at the waist—are more likely to develop heart disease and stroke, even if they have no other risk factors. Excess weight increases the heart's work. It also raises blood pressure, blood cholesterol, and triglyceride levels, and lowers HDL levels. It can also make diabetes more likely to develop. Many overweight people may have difficulty losing weight. But losing even as few as ten pounds can lower your heart disease risk.

Diabetes Mellitus. Diabetes seriously increases your risk of developing cardiovascular disease. Even when glucose (blood sugar) levels are under control, diabetes still increases the risk of heart disease and stroke, but the risks are even greater if blood sugar is not well controlled. About three-quarters of people with diabetes die of some form of heart or blood vessel disease. If you have diabetes, it's extremely important to work with your health care provider to manage it and control any other risk factors you can.

What Are Some Risk Factors That Cannot Be Changed?

Increasing Age. Over 83 percent of people who die of coronary heart disease are 65 or older. At older ages, women who have heart attacks are more likely than men to die from heart disease within a few weeks.

Male Sex (Gender). Men have a greater risk of heart attack than women do, and they have attacks earlier in life. After menopause, women's death rates from heart disease increase significantly, approaching the incidence of men's.

Heredity (Including Race). Children of parents with heart disease are more likely to develop it themselves. African Americans have a greater incidence of severe high blood pressure than Caucasians, as well as a higher risk of heart disease. Heart disease risk is also higher among Mexican Americans, American Indians, native Hawaiians, and some Asian Americans. This is partly due to higher rates of obesity and diabetes. And most people with a strong family history of heart disease have one or more other risk factors.

What Other Factors Can Contribute to Heart Disease Risk?

Stress. Some scientists have noted a relationship between coronary heart disease risk and stress in a person's life, health behaviors, and socioeconomic status. These factors may affect other risk factors. For example, people under stress may overeat, start smoking, or smoke more than they otherwise would.

Drinking. Too much alcohol can raise blood pressure, cause heart failure by directly suppressing heart pumping function, and lead to stroke. It can contribute to high triglycerides, cancer, and other diseases, and produce irregular heartbeats. It contributes to obesity, alcoholism, and suicide.

The risk of heart disease in people who drink moderate amounts of alcohol (an average of one drink for women or two drinks for men per day) may be lower than in nondrinkers. One drink is defined as 1½ fluid ounces of 80-proof spirits (such as bourbon, Scotch, vodka, gin, etc.), 1 fluid ounce of 100-proof spirits, 4 fluid ounces of wine, or 12 fluid ounces of beer. However, it's not recommended that nondrinkers start using alcohol or that drinkers increase the amount they drink. This remains controversial.

Developing a Risk Factor Profile

One quick way to gauge heart attack risk is to look at your family. The presence of obstructive coronary artery disease (significant plaque buildup on the insides of heart artery walls that limit blood flow) in a first-degree relative—parent, brother, sister, or child—age 55 or younger is a significant risk factor for coronary artery disease.

This inherited risk for atherosclerotic heart disease is even more important if the first-degree relative has obstructive coronary artery disease, doesn't smoke, doesn't have diabetes, and is otherwise healthy because that's a strong indication that the heart disease is genetic. So in patients with a prominent family history of premature coronary artery disease, managing the modifiable risk factors takes on even greater importance.

You can determine your risk of experiencing a heart attack by using a risk assessment tool—a ten-year risk calculator—available via the National Heart, Lung, and Blood Institute website. Go to *www.nhlbi.nih.gov/health/index.htm,* and under "Health Assessment Tools" click on "10-Year Heart Attack Risk Calculator."

To use the calculator, you must know your total and high-density lipoprotein cholesterol levels and your systolic blood pressure. Total cholesterol is the sum of all the cholesterol types in your blood. The higher your total cholesterol, the greater your risk of heart disease. High-density lipoprotein is the "good" cholesterol because it picks up cholesterol around the body and carries it through the bloodstream to the liver, which removes it from your system and helps keep cholesterol from accumulating in the walls of arteries. Systolic blood pressure is the measurement of blood pressure during the heart's contraction. It's the first number of the blood pressure reading—for example, the "120" in "120 over 80."

How Does Hypertension Come Into Play?

Hypertension (high blood pressure) is a major risk factor for heart disease and the chief risk factor for stroke and heart failure; it also can lead to kidney damage. Effective hypertension management is crucial to heart disease management. High blood pressure has long been called, and appropriately so, the silent killer because many individuals are unaware of its presence, even when their blood pressure is significantly elevated.

In its early stages, high blood pressure produces no symptoms, so regular physical examinations are important, particularly for anyone with a family history of high blood pressure, heart disease, or diabetes. Physician visits should include blood pressure measurement, prescribing of high blood pressure medications when appropriate (see chapter 5 for more information on blood pressure measurement), and developing strategies for healthy lifestyle changes—quitting smoking, exercising on a regular basis, and losing weight.

Hypertension is also a significant risk factor for atherosclerotic vascular disease. As is the case with atherosclerosis, recent research has led to an improved understanding of hypertension. This new understanding is outlined in the most recent report from the Joint National Committee (JNC) on Prevention, Detection, Evaluation, and Treatment of High Blood Pressure, sometimes referred to as JNC 7 (7 meaning that this is its seventh report).

JNC collects the most recent and best data about hypertension, and then issues guidelines for the prevention, management, and treatment of the condition. (This is known as evidence-based medicine: using evidence—data—to develop guidelines that govern clinical care.) The two most important findings recognized by JNC 7 involve:

- An optimal blood pressure range definition, the range believed most beneficial for maintaining health and avoiding cardiovascular events

- Managing blood pressure with medications

For instance, we know that elevated blood pressure damages arteries, but now we realize that blood pressure levels long considered normal (about 130 over 90 mm Hg for men and for women) may in fact be harmful to arteries.

In 1997, JNC listed six blood pressure categories (optimal, normal, high-normal, and hypertension stages 1, 2, and 3). New research shed new light on blood pressure's effects, so JNC 7 now lists four blood pressure categories (see table below). A new "prehypertension" level accounts for approximately 22 percent of U.S. adults, or about 45 million Americans. The belief is that these tighter blood pressure controls will significantly benefit patients by reducing the risk of cardiovascular and cerebrovascular events.

JNC 7 Blood Pressure Categories

Normal	Prehypertension	Stage 1 HTN	Stage 2 HTN
<120/80 mm Hg	120–139/ 80–89 mm Hg	140–159/ 90–99 mm Hg	<160/100+ mm Hg

HTN = hypertension

Safe management of hypertension involves using medications to *gradually* reduce blood pressure to the optimal range. It's very important, for instance, to avoid dropping your blood pressure too fast, because doing so poses a danger to the brain and other organs by abruptly decreasing their blood supply.

• • • *Fast Fact* • • •

Identifying prehypertension through regular checkups will permit appropriate lifestyle modification efforts to be implemented, often obtaining an optimal blood pressure before medications are required. In fact, it is now recommended that patients with a suspected elevation in blood pressure purchase a home blood pressure monitor. The home monitor permits frequent blood pressure assessments in the home environment, felt to more accurately reflect actual blood pressure as compared to the periodic visit to the physician office, where stress and anxiety can contribute to false blood pressure elevation.

• • •

The JNC 7 guidelines also streamline the steps by which doctors diagnose and treat patients with high blood pressure and recommend the use of diuretics for most patients as part of the initial drug treatment plan.

And in terms of drug therapy, a patient with high blood pressure who has previously had a heart attack will be treated with different medications than will a patient who has, say, hypertension and diabetes. That is because in addition to lowering blood pressure, certain medication classes (beta blockers) have been thoroughly studied and proven to lower heart attack and death rates, for instance, in patients who have suffered a previous heart attack.

Therefore, it's important to educate yourself and consult with your physician as to the best blood pressure-lowering strategy for you.

• • • *Fast Fact* • • •

Diuretics have surprisingly been proven to be excellent first-line agents to treat blood pressure. Why is this surprising? They have been in existence for quite some time plus they are inexpensive. Newer medications with more complex mechanisms of action have been subsequently developed but have not been proven more effective at lowering blood pressure.

• • •

JNC 7 recognizes that prescribing a patient just one blood pressure medication is not often an effective way to keep blood pressure within the optimal range. So if one medication doesn't produce the desired effect, the report recommends using two or possibly three antihypertensive medications to attain blood pressure goals. Since high blood pressure can stem from different problems occurring simultaneously inside the body, it makes sense to use different classes of blood pressure medications to manage the problem. The drugs exert their actions through different pathways, so combining them can produce effective blood pressure control. In clinical circles, this concept is known as synergism: the sum effect from multiple medications is greater than the individual effects.

How Does Hypertension Affect the Heart?

When a person has hypertension, the blood vessels are abnormally constricted, which can significantly increase the heart's workload. The heart is a powerful muscle, but when its workload is increased on a long-term or chronic basis, the muscle can fatigue. This in turn adversely affects blood circulation.

One of the reasons high blood pressure is so dangerous is that, over time, it can lead to congestive heart failure.

In untreated hypertension, the heart's lower chambers, the ventricles, thicken (hypertrophy) and then, over time, enlarge (dilate). The thickening reduces heart compliance. The ventricular tissue stiffens, which results in higher blood pressure inside those lower chambers. This also means the heart doesn't relax the way it's supposed to between heartbeats. The ventricular stiffening can lead to lung congestion, fluid retention, and heart rhythm disturbances. The dilation stretches the ventricular walls, thinning and weakening them. Having lost their ability to contract forcefully, the ventricular walls instead contract sluggishly. In this "hypocontractile" state, the heart's output is reduced, diminishing the delivery of oxygen to the body's tissues and impairing organs' functions. In these later phases of hypertensive heart disease and hypocontractile heart function, congestive heart failure often develops. When this happens, the patient is facing a new set of challenges—a significant deterioration in quality of life, increased risk of death, and, in some extreme cases, the need for heart transplant.

High blood pressure is also associated with atherosclerosis, although how and why this happens isn't fully understood. It's likely that increased stress on the endothelium—the thin inner lining of the blood vessel—creates an environment for atherogenesis: the steady accumulation of fat, cholesterol, platelets, and other blood products beneath the endothelial surface. High blood pressure may contribute to the already turbulent patterns characteristic of blood flow in vessels, particularly where blood vessels branch. This also may disrupt the endothelial lining and promote atherogenesis.

What About Diabetes?

Diabetes mellitus is a chronic condition in which the body is unable to correctly process glucose (sugar), which is used for energy. This disease has no cure. We don't know why, but diabetes increases your risk of developing coronary artery disease and experiencing a cardiovascular event.

What's especially unsettling about diabetes is that, from 2005 to 2007, the Centers for Disease Control and Prevention (CDC) reported that the number of Americans diagnosed increased from 21 to 24 million people, now representing 8 percent of the U.S. population. Although part of the increase is attributed to new methods for recording diagnosed cases, the number of new diabetes cases is markedly rising. Most disturbing of all is that more children are developing the type of diabetes (type 2 or insulin-resistant diabetes) traditionally seen in adults. This means these kids are at risk for developing heart disease. But it's also not surprising because more kids are overweight and even obese, and diabetes is extremely common among overweight people.

Sugar provides energy for cellular function, but it needs help moving from the bloodstream to the inside of a cell. In the body, insulin is the hormone that makes this happen. People with type 1 diabetes do not produce enough insulin; people with type 2 diabetes have inadequate insulin production and their cells resist insulin's action. Provided this insulin resistance, the entry of sugar into cells is at least partially blocked. Importantly, people with diabetes may exhibit atypical atherosclerotic heart disease symptoms, such as shortness of breath, fatigue, and malaise. If they experience chest discomfort, it may be mild rather than severe. Approximately 30 percent of patients with diabetes and advanced coronary artery disease experience no symptoms.

What Is Metabolic Syndrome?

A related condition that is being identified in increasing numbers is metabolic syndrome. The criteria for metabolic syndrome include:

- Insulin resistance
- Elevated waist circumference (abdominal obesity: a waistline greater than 40 inches for men and 35 inches for women)
- Elevated triglyceride levels (more than 150 mg/dL*)
- Low levels of HDL cholesterol (less than 40 mg/dL for men; less than 50 mg/dL for women)
- High blood pressure (more than 130/85 mm Hg†)
- High level of fasting glucose (more than 110 mg/dL)

Metabolic syndrome is of particular concern because people with this condition are at a higher risk for arterial vascular disease. People with metabolic syndrome need to aggressively monitor their blood pressure, diet, physical activities, cholesterol levels, and glucose levels. Such care is best obtained from a clinic or center with diabetes and lipid management expertise. Managing metabolic syndrome must include working with a physician who regularly monitors blood pressure and glucose and cholesterol levels—every three months initially and then every six months. And losing weight is the most helpful thing you can do.

What Are Triglycerides?

A high bloodstream level of serum triglyceride (the chemical form of fat) can cause atherosclerosis and lead to vascular events like heart attacks. Triglycerides serve key roles in the body—for instance, muscles use them for energy—but they're a by-product of ingested dietary fat, absorbed by the gastrointestinal system, and at high levels can be dangerous. Elevated triglycerides are

---

* mg/dL = milligrams per deciliter. Cholesterol levels are measured in milligrams per deciliter of blood.

† mm HG = millimeter of mercury, a unit of pressure.

particularly common in diabetic patients, who also often exhibit the high-risk combination of elevated triglyceride levels and low HDL cholesterol levels.

In addition to taking cholesterol-lowering agents called statins, people with high serum triglyceride levels who do not respond to exercise and changes in diet may also be treated with medications called fibrates or fish oil supplements. This class of medication (fibrates) interferes with triglyceride metabolism and helps the body excrete triglycerides through the bile and into the digestive tract.

Women and Heart Disease

Despite extensive public awareness campaigns, there's still poor awareness about the impact and extent of heart disease on women. Incredibly, heart disease kills more women than breast cancer, yet not enough physicians have educated themselves about heart disease and women. Given that so many heart disease studies have focused on men; that for decades the "male" heart attack has cropped up in movies, books, and television shows; and that "famous" heart attacks—that is, heart attacks that have taken the lives of famous male athletes, entertainers, movie stars, and politicians—dominate the headlines, it's not surprising that heart disease gradually became considered a disease of men.

We discussed some of the key issues regarding heart disease and women in chapter 1, but it's worth revisiting them here. Women and men share the same risk factors for heart disease, but women also have additional risk factors of which they need to be aware. One is menopause. During this time, high blood pressure incidence increases, there's a greater chance for coronary artery disease, and the death rate from heart disease rises. Another factor is race—African-American women are at higher risk for heart disease than women of other races. And when women do develop heart disease, they tend to fare worse than men. Women also tend to

Additional Info

It's important to note that women do not respond as favorably to stenting and bypass grafting procedures with a heightened propensity for stent and bypass graft reblockage. Survival rates for women after a heart attack are less than they are for men. No one knows why this is true, but some have implicated their smaller body mass as a potential reason. Much research is still needed in this area to identify the reasons for and to correct this disparity.

have smaller coronary arteries, which may account for the poorer outcomes in the wake of bypass surgery and stent placement.

There are also subtle differences between women and men with regard to heart disease and heart attack signs and symptoms. In women, some heart disease symptoms can be easily overlooked or mistaken as normal, inconsequential physiological occurrences. These include breathlessness without chest pain; flu-like symptoms (nausea, clamminess); fatigue or weakness; pressure in the lower chest that's mistaken for a stomach ailment; indigestion; pain in the upper back, shoulders, neck, or jaw; and feelings of anxiety (see also chapter 3, page 51 for more about women and heart attack symptoms). Because many women haven't been educated about heart disease, they tend to dismiss these symptoms as unimportant. And clinicians also fail to recognize them as possible signs of heart disease.

Fortunately, efforts are underway to educate women about heart disease. One such effort is The Heart Truth, a national awareness campaign for women spearheaded by the National Heart, Lung, and Blood Institute and other organizations. The campaign's goal is to issue a "wakeup call" to women about their risk of heart disease. Go to *www.nhlbi.nih.gov/health/hearttruth* to learn more about this program.

Nancy's Story

Although she didn't know it at the time, Nancy's heart disease odyssey began in the spring of 1995, at age 40, when she experienced some unsettling episodes of shortness of breath. These aberrant events seemed to arise out of the blue. So Nancy made an appointment to see her primary care physician. At the time, Nancy was "perfectly" healthy—that is, if outward appearance is an accurate indicator of health. She was single and employed as a bank manager, enjoyed an active social life, and was rarely sick.

But she was also a three-pack-a-day smoker (since age 13), a junk-food addict, a workaholic, and she never exercised. Her cholesterol levels would have gotten the attention of the Guinness World Records, if there were such a category.

Nancy's physician ordered an exercise stress test, which can reveal the presence of heart disease. Ironically, Nancy's striking collection of heart disease red flags did not result in a referral to a cardiologist but rather to a pulmonologist, partly because he worked in the same office. Both Nancy's physician and the pulmonologist agreed that the stress-test results were inconclusive, and Nancy did well on the recovery, the phase of the test that monitors the heart's return to a normal rate. Sensing that Nancy's troubles were more likely due to stress, the physicians suggested psychotherapy.

Nancy's instincts, however, told her that something other than stress was causing the problem. At the time, she didn't have the knowledge to connect the risk-factor dots: high blood pressure, chain smoking, poor diet, and one of the most significant risk factors, a rich family history of heart disease. (Her mother had been diagnosed with heart disease and would eventually undergo bypass surgery; her mother's two siblings, a brother and sister, both had undergone bypass surgery; all her mother's first cousins had heart disease. In fact, just about everybody in her mom's family had heart disease.)

It was another few years before Nancy went in for reassessment, this time with her mother's primary care physician and again spurred by a shortness-of-breath episode. But nothing much came of that office visit either. By that time, Nancy was getting used to the shortness-of-breath episodes, so she was less concerned.

Then, one day in February 1999, Nancy began having chest pains. That symptom was a major call for help from her heart, which had a dangerously narrowed artery. Nancy's physician immediately set her up with Holter monitoring, which provides a continuous recording of heart rhythm during normal activity over twenty-four hours. The results showed twenty-five episodes of ST segment depressions, sure signs of developing heart attack. Nancy was told to see a cardiologist right away.

• • • *Fast Fact* • • •

Holter monitoring is at present rarely used to assess for heart artery blockages. It has been supplanted by cardiac imaging with stress testing being the current mainstay.

• • •

That's when things got tricky. Nancy was admitted to her local hospital's cardiology department, where the physicians quickly determined she needed a catheterization to give a clearer idea about the source of the problem. But that wasn't going to be easy. A good number of the city's cardiologists were in New Orleans at the time, attending an annual international heart meeting. A catheterization team wouldn't be available until the following day. "We'll keep you overnight," they said. But Nancy was feeling antsy. She wasn't keen on spending a night in the hospital. So she left with a prescription for nitroglycerin and an appointment early the next morning with an interventional cardiology team.

A good friend, who happened to work in the electrophysiology lab at a nearby hospital, had been monitoring Nancy's odyssey that day. When she heard about the situation with the "cath" team, she too got antsy. "I'm coming over there to pick up a copy of your EKG. I want someone here to see it," she insisted. Shortly thereafter, Nancy's cousin drove her to the drugstore to have the nitroglycerin prescription filled. While Nancy was inside, her cell phone started ringing. Her cousin sensed the call was important, so she answered the phone. It was Dr. T., calling from the Cleveland Clinic's Department of Cardiovascular Medicine. The cousin explained that Nancy was unavailable. "I'll wait," said Dr. T. When Nancy got back in the car, her cousin handed her the cell phone. "It's the Cleveland Clinic calling," she said.

Nancy listened to Dr. T. make his case. "I've looked at your EKG results. Now, it makes no difference to me which hospital does the catheterization. What's most important, however, is that you are in a hospital, so that you can be monitored and get on a nitroglycerin drip. So I really think you should get down here right away."

The phone call, and the insistence in Dr. T.'s voice, got Nancy's attention. Her cousin drove her down to the Clinic, where she was admitted, stayed overnight, and underwent catheterization the next morning. Findings showed 95 percent narrowing of the left anterior descending artery, one of the heart's main vessels, and 40 percent blockage in the right coronary artery. The right coronary artery could be managed with medications and lifestyle changes, but the left coronary artery needed angioplasty and stenting.

Aftermath

Heart disease changed Nancy's life. The chain-smoking has been replaced with exercise, the junk food with a heart-healthy diet. She takes a statin every day. For friends and colleagues who remember her as the workaholic whose hand always held a burning cigarette—who, in fact, often had two or three cigarettes burning at once—the change is dramatic.

The same tenacity and discipline that characterizes Nancy's professional life now also fuels her mission to stay healthy. She exercises regularly and is ruthless about maintaining a healthy diet. Now in her 50s, she's in top physical shape. The lifestyle changes toppled her bad cholesterol levels. Prior to the angioplasty and stenting, she had a total cholesterol of 250 mg/dL and an LDL of 172! (The recommended LDL range today is less than 100 mg/dL.) Her HDL, the good cholesterol, was in the 30s. (The recommended HDL range today is 55 mg/dL or higher.) The hard work, discipline, smoking cessation, and medical therapy essentially flipped things. By 2005, she had her LDL down to 53 mg/dL and HDL up to 110 mg/dL. That's quite a turnaround.

But as Nancy explains it, there was incentive to make changes. "I decided that if I wanted to stay alive, I'd have to do everything I could to get healthy and stay healthy. My mom and all of her relatives had heart disease in their 50s and 60s. And I'm diagnosed in my 40s. So I started exercising. I went to cardiac rehab three days a week for a year, most of which I paid for myself because insurance doesn't cover the second phase of the program. I changed my diet. I cut out fats, sweets, all the bad stuff. Now, everything is low-fat. All the restaurants I visit frequently know I only eat low-fat. Grilled fish, no oil, no butter, steamed vegetables, sushi, chicken, turkey. And I haven't touched beef since June 2003."

Like many smokers, Nancy had made countless promises to herself about quitting. "It bothered me at age 20 that I smoked," she says. She kept promising to quit "next year." Then, as the years went by, "I kept thinking, I'll be able to quit smoking before it does something to physically harm me. I always thought I'd be able to do that." She promised to quit again and again. "But I never gave myself a deadline. It was just like 'Yeah, I'll do it.'"

The fear of death, however, put her situation into perspective. And rather than attempt some sort of gradual weaning, she decided to go cold turkey. "Quitting was hard. Every day for the first year, I counted the number of days I had quit. But after that first year, it got easier."

Today, Nancy is thriving and healthy. Her passion about staying healthy and educating other women about heart disease led to volunteer efforts with the local chapter of the American Heart Association. She now sits on its board.

Overcoming the Risks

We can reduce among women the death rate from heart disease, but women must become proactive about educating themselves and their doctors. This means getting familiar with one's family history, learning how to live a heart-healthy life, and engaging your physician in a conversation about heart disease. And women need to be proactive about seeing a physician on a regular basis.

This is particularly the case since a bias still exists concluding that women are protected against developing heart disease. Nothing can be further from the truth. Especially important is heart disease prevention in women. As I have outlined, once a woman develops coronary artery disease, the stakes are even higher as women do not respond as well to revascularization procedures plus they possess lower heart attack survival rates compared to men. We as a healthcare community are making progress in leveling this playing field but further inroads are needed. I am confident, over time, that the various campaigns highlighting the importance of heart disease in women will have the two-fold result of both patient and healthcare professional education making a positive difference in heart disease incidence rates and outcomes amongst women.

Chapter 5

Heart Health Assessment

The heart health assessment is a thorough examination designed to identify heart disease risk factors, existing heart problems, or previously undiagnosed conditions like high blood pressure. The heart health assessment is the cardiologist's means of determining one's overall heart health.

An effective and thorough heart health assessment consists of four essential steps:

- Obtaining a patient history
- Performing a physical exam
- Drawing blood for laboratory testing
- Measuring the heart's electrical activity in individuals suspected of having heart disease or heart problems utilizing electrocardiography

When appropriate, heart health assessment can involve performing additional testing, such as exercise stress testing and a cardiac ultrasound known as an echocardiogram. These tests further assess heart function and identify the potential for disease.

A detailed patient history involves asking a broad range of questions about your family's health, your health, smoking history (if any), diet, level of physical activity or exercise, whether you're experiencing possible heart disease symptoms that warrant further investigation, whether you're taking medications, and, if so, for what conditions. This information, along with your age and weight, will be used to ascertain risk factors and to make calculations about heart attack risk. Risk factors (see chapter 4) include smoking, being overweight, sedentary lifestyle, diabetes, hypertension, and family history of heart disease.

What Is a Physical Heart Health Exam Like?

Here's what my exam typically is like: I record your vital signs (temperature, pulse, rate of breathing, blood pressure) and may also measure the blood pressure in your ankle and arm (ankle-brachial testing), palpate (feel) pulses at different points on the body, and use a stethoscope to listen to your lungs, heart, and the major arteries. Although the initial physical exam uses fundamental, noninvasive assessment techniques, it can provide telling information.

Placing a stethoscope bell on, above, or near one of the major arteries—like the carotid, which courses through the neck and up into the brain to deliver oxygenated blood—I listen for any abnormal sound indicative of turbulent blood flow. A whooshing sound—known as a bruit (pronounced "brew-ee")—emanating from one of these sources may signal a carotid artery problem that requires further investigation. By placing the stethoscope bell at various points on your torso, I can check for irregular sounds emanating from the heart, such as a "murmur" caused by a bad heart valve, or an extra heart sound indicative of heart muscle stiffening and/or weakening.

Some heart murmurs are innocent; some are suspect. The innocent ones are called functional murmurs and indicate the normal acceleration of blood flow through the cardiac chambers. Suspect

The Ankle-Brachial Index

The ankle-brachial index (ABI) is an important source of information. An abnormal ABI may be the first sign of arterial vascular disease; it's also a powerful predictor of arterial vascular events, such as heart attacks and strokes.

In this simple blood pressure test, a cuff is placed around the upper arm and then the upper leg. The readings are compared, and if the numbers are greatly different, peripheral arterial blockage is suspected.

or abnormal heart murmurs indicate a leaking or abnormally narrowed heart valve.

Checking for abdominal aortic enlargement is also important. This involves palpating the abdomen and attempting to gauge the width of the aorta by feeling its pulsation. If an aneurysm is present, the pulse may be exaggerated, diffuse, and less pinpoint, compared to normal. Palpation, however, particularly in overweight individuals, is often an ineffective way to judge aortic size. When aortic enlargement is suspected, a better alternative is an imaging tool such as a vascular ultrasound. Computed tomography (CT) and magnetic resonance imaging (MRI) also provide precise aortic imaging. Unlike vascular ultrasound, both require an intravenous line and the injection of an imaging agent. CT also involves ionizing radiation exposure.

What Kind of Lab Tests Can I Expect as Part of a Heart Health Assessment?

Cardiac laboratory testing often involves analyzing blood to measure lipid levels, and the resulting report is called a lipid panel. It provides information about your levels of good and bad cholesterol (HDL-C and LDL-C, respectively) as well as triglycerides. These lipid measures are terms that you've likely heard many times, but most people don't know exactly what they mean or exactly what the recommended ranges are, so I've included a table from the American Heart Association that helps sort this out. Keep in mind that a lipid panel is just one component of a heart health assessment and that the ranges for cholesterol and triglycerides are just that—ranges.

Certainly, a finding that's remarkably high or low warrants attention. But there's no reason to panic if lipid panel results don't exactly match the recommended ranges. Also, other factors—for instance, a family history *free* of heart disease—weigh in your favor when a lipid panel finding is out of the recommended range. But this equation works both ways. Smokers should not assume all is well just because lipid panel results show nothing remarkable.

Another blood test often ordered measures the level of lipoprotein (a), a type of low-density lipoprotein. Lipoproteins are particles that circulate in your blood, and a high reading indicates a heightened risk of atherosclerosis. Even with an improved diet and exercise program, elevated lipoprotein (a) levels are difficult to treat. Existing medications exert a modest lowering effect.

Cholesterol Guidelines. Initial classification based on total cholesterol and HDL cholesterol:

Total Cholesterol Level	Category
Less than 200 mg/dL	Desirable level that puts you at lower risk for coronary heart disease. A cholesterol level of 200 mg/dL or higher raises your risk.
200–239 mg/dL	Borderline high.
240 mg/dL and above	High blood cholesterol. A person with this level has more than twice the risk of coronary heart disease of someone whose cholesterol is below 200 mg/dL.

HDL Cholesterol Level	Category
Less than 40 mg/dL (for men) Less than 50 mg/dL (for women)	Low HDL cholesterol. A major risk factor for heart disease.
60 mg/dL and above	High HDL cholesterol. An HDL of 60 mg/dL above is considered protective against heart disease.

If your total cholesterol is 200 mg/dL or more, or your HDL cholesterol is less than 40 mg/dL, you need to have a lipoprotein profile done to determine your LDL cholesterol and triglyceride levels. If your cholesterol is high or you have other risk factors, your health-care provider will likely want to monitor your cholesterol levels more closely. Follow your provider's advice about how often to have your cholesterol tested. He or she will set appropriate management goals based on your LDL cholesterol level and other risk factors.

LDL Cholesterol Level	Category
Less than 100 mg/dL	Optimal
100–129 mg/dL	Near or above optimal
130–159 mg/dL	Borderline high
160–189 mg/dL	High
190 mg/dL and above	Very high

Your LDL cholesterol goal depends on how many other risk factors you have.

- If you don't have coronary heart disease or diabetes, and have one or no risk factors, your LDL goal is less than 160 mg/dL.

- If you don't have coronary heart disease or diabetes, and have two or more risk factors, your LDL goal is less than 130 mg/dL.

- If you do have coronary heart disease or diabetes, your LDL goal is less than 100 mg/dL.

Triglyceride is the most common type of fat in the body. Many people who have heart disease or diabetes have high triglyceride levels. Normal triglyceride levels vary by age and gender. A high triglyceride level combined with low HDL cholesterol or high LDL cholesterol seems to speed up atherosclerosis. Atherosclerosis increases the risk for heart attack and stroke.

Triglyceride Level*	Category
Less than 150 mg/dL	Normal
150–199 mg/dL	Borderline high
200–499 mg/dL	High
500 mg/dL and above	Very high

• • • *Fast Fact* • • •

In patients with established arterial vascular disease, it's recommended that the LDL cholesterol level be less than 70 mg/dL and the total cholesterol level less than 150 mg/dL. In terms of arterial vascular disease, there's no such thing as levels that are too low. My practice is to set a goal of extremely low cholesterol levels in these patients, most typically through the use of high-dose statins and careful and frequent blood sample monitoring.

• • •

---

* Triglyceride Level Chart reproduced with permission American Heart Association, *www.americanheart.org* ©2006, American Heart Association.

Biomarkers. Depending on your family and medical history, your blood also may be tested for certain cardiac biomarkers—molecules found in the bloodstream that can provide important information about the status of atherosclerosis. A biomarker could be one of several kinds of molecules—an enzyme, protein, or hormone. Just as we measure cholesterol levels, we do the same for these bio-markers. Depending on the situation, a biomarker can be used to confirm the existence of disease or provide information about the extent of its progression.

Today, one of the most revealing biomarkers is the ultrasensitive C-reactive protein (US-CRP), also known as high-sensitivity

Red Flag

Ultrasensitive C-reactive protein is assuming even greater promi-nence. A recent study measured ultrasensitive C-reactive protein levels in patients with normal cholesterol levels. Patients were assigned to two groups, one group receiving statins and the other a placebo (a sugar pill). The study was terminated prematurely as those patients with normal serum lipid parameters and an elevated ultrasensitive C-reactive protein level that were admin-istered statins demonstrated significantly lower heart attack and cardiac death rates. This study highlights the complexity of treat-ing coronary atherosclerosis and the fact that cholesterol levels are not the sole predeterminants for atherosclerotic heart disease events. The role of vascular inflammation cannot be overstated. Atherosclerotic vascular disease is an extremely dynamic process with heightened cellular activity including rapid cell manufacturing and turnover. While the exact mechanism of the favorable impact of statins on event rates is not known, it is believed with reason-able confidence that this cellular activity is diminished, which in part contributes to the conversion of soft and potentially unstable plaque to hard and more stable plaques, less prone to fissuring, rupture, and abrupt blood clot formation.

C-reactive protein. People with high levels of this protein are thought to have a high degree of inflammation at atherosclerotic sites and are believed to experience a greater likelihood of vascular events, such as heart attack and stroke. Statins can successfully lower CRP levels; exercise and weight loss also appear to help keep high CRP levels in check. Testing for US-CRP is inexpensive, and the results are instructive to the patient and physician.

Blood Pressure Measurement. It's really never too early to begin monitoring blood pressure. Ideally, blood pressure should be checked annually—and more frequently when a strong family history of hypertension or heart disease is evident.

Obtaining an accurate blood pressure measurement is easy as long as the proper techniques are used and the blood pressure monitoring equipment is functioning accurately. But people need to understand that a onetime measurement during an office visit isn't an effective means of getting a clear picture of an individual's blood pressure profile, and it shouldn't be the basis for the initiation of any therapy until results are repeated and confirmed.

There is one exception—when the blood pressure is excessively high (e.g., 220/120 mm Hg). This isn't normal, even in a person exhibiting significant anxiety, and it merits treatment with medication *at the time of the office visit.* If urgency warrants it, particularly with symptoms of shortness of breath, chest discomfort, a severe headache, or perceived visual changes, a short hospital stay may be prudent. (The goal, however, is to lower blood pressure gradually; we're not trying to achieve same-day results. In fact, we want to avoid same-day results. The body actually acclimates to high blood pressure, so lowering it in a matter of hours is risky—doing so could result in a dangerous reduction of blood flow to vital areas, especially the brain.)

In emergencies, the initial blood pressure measurement provides vital information that guides clinical action. But in these situations, measurements are taken many times over the course of emergency management.

The bottom line: effective, accurate blood pressure monitoring and the confident diagnosis of hypertension involve a series of at least three measurements obtained on different days. One strategy, although not very convenient, is a series of weekly office visits spread over a period of three to four weeks. If your physician is not available, these appointments can be scheduled with nurses, who subsequently forward the blood pressure measurements to your doctor in aggregate for interpretation and treatment recommendations.

Under normal circumstances, blood pressure rises and falls throughout the day in tune with the body's natural circadian rhythms; it's also lower at night and higher during the day. And caffeine intake, eating certain foods, smoking, physical activity, illness, anxiety, and stress affect blood pressure. Since blood pressure may be higher or lower depending on the time of day, a onetime measurement provides an inadequate picture of your blood pressure profile. So blood pressure measurements should be taken at variable times throughout the day to get a good sense of your health.

Some people get nervous in a doctor's office. So even if they have normal blood pressure, their measurement at that moment may suggest otherwise. Clinicians call this effect "white coat hypertension"—that is, elevated blood pressure in the presence of a physician ("white coat") or another healthcare worker.

Patients should be relaxed, seated in a comfortable chair, and the arm should be supported in some way, with the forearm horizontal and the elbow at 45 degrees. A blood pressure cuff should never be wrapped around clothing; rolling up sleeves is not a good means of freeing the arm. Patients should be seated for several minutes before a blood pressure cuff is placed on an arm, and two, rather than one, blood pressure measurements should be taken;

ideally, this should occur in each arm, several minutes apart. Why both arms? Because blood pressure in one arm can be significantly lower than the other. When this happens, it's generally a signal of obstructive atherosclerosis. Most often, this involves one of the two subclavian arteries, large vessels sprouting from the aorta; these arteries course from the aorta to the right and left arms to deliver oxygenated blood.

Every time a patient seeks medical care, blood pressure should be measured; in fact, this occurs in most medical settings in the United States. Keeping a blood pressure monitor at home—automatic devices can be purchased at drugstores and pharmacies—is also a good idea for proactive monitoring in people at risk for or who have been diagnosed with high blood pressure, heart disease, or diabetes.

Patients with either suspect or poorly controlled blood pressure should be measured daily, with the results recorded in a blood pressure log or diary that can be shared with their physician every month. Once the blood pressure target is reached, blood pressure monitoring can occur every few days. For some patients, particularly those just starting blood pressure control with medications, measurements should be taken in the morning and evening. The results from twice-daily measurements can help the prescribing

Please Note

In my experience, when I have my blood pressure checked, the biggest error I observe is that the cuff is not inflated high enough to ensure accurate recording of the top number or systolic blood pressure. The second most common error is when the cuff is deflated too quickly, resulting in blood pressure numbers that are estimates and not accurate measurements. This is completely avoidable by doing careful work in a systematic and nonrushed manner. As a patient, do your best to ensure that this is the case.

Red Flag

Should you purchase a home blood pressure monitor, which I do recommend, make sure you speak with your physician regarding the brand and model that he might suggest. Not all products are of similar quality and therefore accuracy. Do not pinch pennies with this purchase. Also, once you purchase your new monitor, make sure that you take it to your doctor's office to have its accuracy checked against their more sophisticated equipment. If it is off by a few millimeters of mercury, that's okay and you can add or subtract the difference from your readings at home and record your numbers accordingly. If it is off by ten points or more, consider returning your monitor for an alternative brand or model. I also encourage my patients to bring their monitor with them to each visit. That way we can check the accuracy of their home equipment over time.

A number of years ago I decided to provide my email address to my patients. One of the principle reasons that I did this was for my patients to send their monthly blood pressure logs to me for my review. This way, with a home machine that both the patient and I trust, we together can stay on top of their blood pressure frequently, adjusting medication types and doses as needed.

physician make appropriate decisions about dosing (including at what time of day a blood pressure drug should be taken), adding a drug, or switching from one to another, to optimize blood pressure control and to minimize side effects.

Ambulatory Blood Pressure Monitoring. Effective, accurate blood pressure monitoring involves a series of measurements taken over several weeks or multiple measurements recorded over a short period, using a special portable device that automatically documents blood pressure levels. This is called ambulatory blood pressure monitoring.

In ambulatory monitoring, a blood pressure cuff that's secured to the upper arm is connected by wires to a small recording device that hangs from a belt strapped around the waist. The apparatus records blood pressure at regular intervals during a twenty-four-hour period. This method has proven to be quite accurate in assessing blood pressure over a longer period of time.

Readings produced by ambulatory blood pressure monitoring can reveal at what points during a twenty-four-hour period blood pressure is highest and lowest, as well as what a person's average blood pressure is over that period. For patients on blood pressure medications, ambulatory monitoring shows when, throughout the day, blood pressure is being controlled. It also reveals systolic and diastolic values. For patients prone to white coat hypertension and for whom self-monitoring of blood pressure is not an option, ambulatory monitoring is an invaluable alternative. So this is a very important tool for obtaining detailed information about high blood pressure and how well it's being medically managed.

As discussed above, another option is monitoring your blood pressure at home with an automatic sphygmomanometer, which can be purchased at a pharmacy or large retailer. The device lets you measure your blood pressure on a regular basis; record the findings; and fax, email, or bring them to follow-up office visits.

How Is My Heart's Electrical Activity Measured?

Electrocardiogram Testing. An electrocardiogram (EKG, also known as ECG) records the heart's electrical activity from the chest wall surface. It provides information on the heart rate and heart rhythm, cardiac chamber position and size, and heart muscle thickness. It can also identify acute heart attacks, reveal evidence of a prior but undiagnosed heart attack, and help identify where on the heart's surface the heart attack damage has occurred. The electrocardiogram is often used to assess the benefit of cardiac medications, especially those targeting abnormal heart rhythms; it can also record the surface electrical activity of devices such as implanted pacemakers. It is an ideal test—it is quick and inexpensive to administer, produces no discomfort or risk, and yields a wealth of immediate information.

The EKG collects information via ten wires or leads placed at six precise locations across the center and left portion of the chest and also attached to each extremity. The test records the heart's electrical activity (the electrical current running through the heart) and prints out findings that you can discuss with your physician.

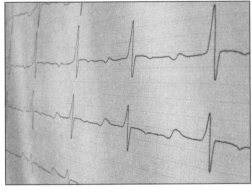

If you undergo EKG testing, request a copy of the test results. Take the results to a photocopy machine, make a reduced wallet-sized version of the tracing, and laminate it and carry it with you at all times. Should an emergency arise, that EKG reading can be compared with any new electrocardiogram changes, which can help physicians unfamiliar with your medical history to make facilitated clinical decisions on your behalf with greater accuracy.

The Stress Test

A stress test is a noninvasive (external) means of assessing your coronary artery circulation. In other words, it provides information about how well the heart reacts to an increased oxygen demand. If you had to pick just one test for determining the likelihood of a future cardiac event, the exercise stress test, with its ability to measure exercise capacity, oxygen use, and heart rate recovery, is one of the best diagnostic tests in cardiovascular medicine.

A stress test can diagnose the presence of coronary artery disease or monitor patients with preexisting coronary artery disease. Stress testing takes two forms—exercise and nonexercise. The latter also is known as pharmacological stress testing.

To maximize the information produced during a stress test, it is combined with continuous electrocardiogram monitoring and intermittent blood pressure monitoring. EKG information is obtained during the rest and exercise modes of the stress test. (Stress testing also can be combined with echocardiography or nuclear imaging, both of which produce images of the heart.)

Exercise stress testing involves a walk on a treadmill or a "ride" on a stationary bicycle under the supervision of clinicians. The test's objective is to reach an age-adjusted predetermined heart rate, so the length of the test depends in part on how the heart responds. The exercise pace is gradually increased until the target heart rate is reached. However, if EKG or blood pressure monitoring reveals abnormalities, testing will be stopped.

Exercise stress testing is used to identify myocardial ischemia (oxygen deprivation of heart muscle). Basically, stress testing allows cardiologists to gauge your heart's "tolerance" for physical activity.

Myocardial ischemia generally occurs when coronary artery atherosclerosis obstructs more than 70 percent of the cross-sectional blood flow in a vessel. But ischemia arises only during physical exertion unless an artery is critically narrowed, generally 90 percent or greater in the cross-sectional area. Physical activity increases blood pressure and the pulse rate because the body's demand for oxygenated blood increases. That means the heart has to work harder, but it also means the heart itself requires an increased supply of oxygenated blood. A coronary artery with significant narrowing can't meet the demand of the heart muscle cells it serves—it can't deliver enough oxygenated blood fast enough. When heart cells don't receive enough oxygenated blood, the heart's pumping capacity is reduced. So by inducing ischemia, stress testing can reveal significant coronary artery narrowing.

Stopping the physical activity reduces the burden on the heart and will return heart function to normal when oxygen supply to the heart muscle and oxygen demand of the heart muscle are once again in balance.

A stress test may be recommended if you:

- Possess a strong family history of premature coronary artery disease

- Are a sedentary person interested in beginning an exercise program, particularly if you have multiple heart attack risk factors such as a family history of heart disease, smoking, overweight, high blood pressure, diabetes, or a recent episode of chest pain

- Have documented atherosclerosis and are scheduled for major noncardiac vascular surgery, such as an abdominal aortic aneurysm repair

- Experience unexplained chest discomfort

- Have experienced an uncomplicated heart attack (one with no symptoms/signs of congestive heart failure or recurrent chest discomfort) and remain ambulatory with a preserved exercise capacity

Exercise stress testing can also check blood flow in a vessel that has undergone angioplasty and/or stenting. The results reveal how open the vessel is. When you hear cardiologists use the term *patency*, they're referring to openness in an artery that has undergone intervention to widen it.

What Does the Stress Test Reveal About My Blood Pressure Response?

An important parameter during an exercise stress test is the blood pressure response. A normal blood pressure response is characterized by a gradual increase in systolic blood pressure (the blood pressure during a heart contraction). At the highest level of exertion, systolic pressure might range from the high 100s or low 200s mm Hg. But if after the initial increase in systolic pressure, blood pressure plateaus or *decreases* at still higher levels of exertion, exercise-induced heart dysfunction—where the heart can't meet the oxygen demands of the body's organs and tissues—might be present. This imbalance often signals the presence of significant coronary artery disease.

Before an exercise stress test is administered, we use various pieces of information, including age and general fitness level, to determine an optimal exercise schedule and target heart rate. The target heart rate is the number of heartbeats per minute your heart needs to achieve during a diagnostic test. A result from an exercise test during which the target heart rate is achieved (a diagnostic test) is considered more accurate than one from a test during which the target is not achieved (a nondiagnostic test). The latter, when normal, cannot be completely trusted in terms of the absence of flow-limiting coronary artery disease as it was a submaximal test with an inadequate attained heart rate.

During the stress test, the EKG allows for continuous monitoring of the heart's electrical activity. Blood pressure measurement at regular intervals provides up-to-the-minute information about the cardiovascular response to exercise. This ensures that we quickly identify signs or symptoms that warrant stopping the testing or easing up the exercise pace so that unwanted complications such as heart rhythm abnormalities or abnormally high blood pressure can be avoided.

A healthy patient will hit the exercise test target heart rate. What warrants further investigation are significant arrhythmias, hypotension (abnormally low blood pressure), and abnormal electrocardiogram findings that are discovered during exercise testing.

An exercise stress test, which achieves a higher rate pressure product and places a higher level of stress on the heart, is always preferable to nonexercise forms of stress testing. The rate pressure product is defined as the maximal pulse rate, in beats per minute, multiplied by the maximal systolic blood pressure, attained during exercise testing. With exercise, these values are typically much higher and therefore result in a greater level of stress on the heart compared to the nonexercise form of stress testing.

• • • *Fast Fact* • • •

This does not mean that nonexercise stress testing does not provide value. On the contrary, nonexercise stress tests possess an excellent track record for identifying previously undiagnosed obstructive coronary artery disease. It's just that regular exercise provides more parameters to assess and draw a more confident conclusion such as exercise duration, the rapidity of the pulse rate recovery after exercise, and also the blood pressure response to exercise. These parameters are either not measurable or less meaningful with nonexercise forms of stress testing.

• • •

Will the Stress Test Gauge How Physically Fit I Am?

Exercise stress testing allows cardiologists to accurately assess a person's overall fitness (also known as peak performance or exercise capacity). Peak performance—the highest level of exercise you are capable of achieving during a treadmill exercise test—is expressed in units of metabolic equivalents (METS). This is a measure of oxygen use per kilogram of body weight per minute.

A high fitness level is characterized by a METS value in the range of 14.0 to 16.0; a poor fitness level is a METS value in the range of 1.0 to 3.9. The higher the METS result achieved, the less likely you are to experience a cardiovascular event. For example, advanced multivessel coronary artery obstructions often result in profound myocardial ischemia, blunting the exercise capacity typically associated with a submaximal METS value.

Another important exercise stress testing parameter is heart rate recovery. That's the rate at which your pulse returns to "baseline" after you stop exercising. Baseline refers to the heart rate (number of beats per minute) maintained when you aren't exercising and are relaxed. Under optimal conditions, the heart rate should return to its baseline fairly soon—within several minutes—after exercise ceases. For a healthy adult, this means the heart rate decreases by eighteen or more beats during the first minute after exercise stops. In general, a normal heart rate recovery equates with a favorable cardiovascular prognosis.

What Is an Abnormal Stress Test Response?

Abnormal clinical responses during exercise stress testing include chest pain, significant increases or decreases in blood pressure, and the inability to exercise longer than three minutes before stopping.

Patients who exhibit significant heart rhythm disorders (called arrhythmias) during stress testing are at higher risk for future heart rhythm disturbances. Finding an arrhythmia can signal, for example, the presence of obstructive coronary artery disease (plaque buildup in an artery that impedes blood flow), structural heart disease such as heart muscle weakening or thickening, or valvular heart disease.

Additionally, ST segment depression, an abnormal electrocardiogram finding, suggests the presence of obstructive coronary artery disease. In individuals with significant obstructive coronary disease, the exercise electrocardiogram will correctly reflect the problem 65 to 70 percent of the time, and this is visible in the form of depressed ST segments on the EKG strip.

In a patient with normal coronary arteries, we see normal ST segments approximately 70 percent of the time, meaning that

30 percent of the time we're getting a misleading or "false positive" finding. That's why cardiac imaging is used in conjunction with EKG stress testing—it improves diagnostic accuracy. In fact, the imaging finding often supersedes the electrocardiogram finding when ascribing an overall interpretation to the stress test.

Cardiac imaging further improves the diagnostic accuracy of exercise stress testing so it's widely used in cardiac diagnostic testing. Echocardiography (not to be confused with *electro*cardiography, which measures electrical activity) and nuclear imaging (often referred to as nuclear stress testing) of the heart also can be combined with pharmacological, or nonexercise, stress testing.

What Is Echocardiography?

Echocardiogram stress testing uses ultrasound technology, via an echocardiography machine, to produce a live image of the heart. Much the same way ultrasonography produces real-time images of a fetus, echocardiography produces images of the heart and nearby structures. In this procedure, a probe placed on the patient's chest provides a wealth of information about the heart, including the strength of heart muscle contraction, evidence of prior heart attack(s), valvular function, cardiac chamber size, and heart wall thickness. It also provides information about surrounding cardiac structures, including the sac around the heart (pericardium).

When echocardiography accompanies stress testing, imaging of the heart occurs before exercise, when the patient is still resting, and immediately after exercise, when the target or peak exercise heart rate is still present. Comparing the pre-exercise and postexercise images side by side in a digitized computer format permits a detailed examination of heart wall motion so cardiologists can detect significant coronary artery obstructions ("significant" meaning that an artery lumen has narrowed by 70 percent or more).

Echocardiography reveals any heart wall abnormalities. When heart muscle receives an adequate supply of oxygenated blood, it responds appropriately when the body asks it to pump harder and faster. This is called a hypercontractile response, and it's characterized in part by thickening of the tissue as it contracts to pump blood. When the blood supply is inadequate because of a narrowed artery, a hypocontractile response occurs: the tissue doesn't thicken or contract adequately. If more than one artery with plaque blockage interferes with blood flow, the problem is compounded because now two or more "territories" of heart muscle can't get enough oxygenated blood during physical exertion. Echocardiography can reveal this hypocontractile behavior that arises during exercise stress testing. As with any stress testing, be it echocardiography or nuclear medicine based, an abnormality suggesting obstructive coronary artery disease typically culminates in further evaluation by performing a cardiac catheterization.

What Is Nuclear Stress Testing?

Nuclear stress testing involves injecting a "tracer" into the bloodstream about one minute before the exercise stress test ends. In this case, the tracer is a radioactive substance (isotope), and the two most commonly used for exercise testing are thallium and technetium. Tracers are given in very small amounts and don't harm the body. Once injected, tracers travel quickly through the bloodstream to the heart and, via the coronary arteries, concentrate in the heart muscle. They also emit rays that can be detected by an imaging device called a gamma camera.

In general, the patient undergoes gamma imaging prior to the exercise test and almost immediately after test completion. (The protocols can vary from one heart center to the next.) For the imaging portion of the test, the patient lays supine on a platform adjacent to the gamma camera.

Please Note

Irrespective of the nuclear medicine stress testing protocol, the key is to obtain pictures of the coronary artery circulation at rest and immediately after exercise. Comparing these sets of pictures provides valuable coronary artery blood flow information at peak cardiac stress.

The emission of the rays by the tracers helps create a "map of cardiac perfusion." In other words, the tracers light up all the areas of the heart that are receiving blood. The darker portions of the image mark areas of the heart that have an inadequate supply of blood or that have been damaged by previous heart attack.

If heart muscle perfusion is normal at rest but abnormal during exercise, this is a strong indication of myocardial ischemia, which is an inadequate supply of blood to the heart tissue. If imaging reveals abnormal heart muscle perfusion at rest and during exercise, this is a sign of heart muscle scarring caused by heart attack.

Interestingly, nuclear stress testing can be unreliable when used on individuals who have diffuse coronary artery disease (this is characterized by multiple arteries in the heart with plaque obstructions, which can prevent adequate blood flow during exertion). In the presence of diffuse coronary artery disease, there's almost an even or balanced reduction of blood flow throughout the heart. This undercuts the tracers' ability to create contrasting (heterogeneous) blood flow patterns, which help mark areas of cardiac tissue with a poor blood supply. Thankfully, such cases are uncommon. Moreover, the exercise electrocardiogram, an assessment of exertional capacity, and echocardiography are fairly effective at identifying the presence of advanced diffuse coronary artery disease when a nuclear stress test is inconclusive.

What Can You Do to Supplement the Nuclear Stress Testing?

Clearly, nuclear stress testing comes with some limitations. As noted, it may not detect diffuse coronary artery disease. It can sometimes overestimate the extent of coronary artery narrowing. A more accurate, sensitive alternative involves positron emission tomography (PET) scanning. Using a PET scan with stress testing is called cardiac PET scanning.

A PET scanner is a doughnut-shaped machine; like nuclear imaging, it produces images from a small amount of radioactive tracer that is "tagged" (attached) to a type of glucose called F-deoxyglucose, which is injected into the bloodstream. Cells rely on glucose for normal function and metabolism. So in cardiac PET scanning, the injected glucose enters heart cells that are alive including those with preserved contractile properties as well as those that are alive but with reduced pumping capacity, so-called viable myocardium. The scanner detects and records the energy given off by the tracers and, with the aid of a computer, converts the energy into three-dimensional pictures. Since the glucose is tagged, it marks the location of metabolically alive tissue. Areas that show no sign of the tagged glucose are considered irreversibly damaged and not likely to benefit from myocardial revascularization in the form of stent placement or coronary artery bypass grafting.

The most commonly used coronary artery blood flow tracer for cardiac PET scanning is rubidium, a material similar to thallium and technetium, the tracers used for traditional nuclear stress testing.

Because PET technology can produce better resolution than nuclear scanning, the resulting images provide a clearer, more accurate picture of cardiac blood flow and how it's affected by artery narrowing or tissue damage from heart attack. Not surprisingly, cardiac PET scanning is more expensive and not widely available. Also, it's not used in combination with exercise stress testing; rather, it's used solely during pharmacological stress testing.

PET scan results can be extremely helpful in assessing patients with reduced heart function due to heart attack. The infarct (destroyed tissue) caused by heart attack often includes a zone of muscle that may still be "alive"—viable myocardium—but with echocardiography appears dysfunctional or "sleepy." By viable, cardiologists mean that with effective intervention that restores blood flow, this heart muscle tissue has the potential to regain near-normal function, even months or years after the damage has occurred. So it's very important to be able to identify this potentially viable tissue. The key is to identify weakened heart muscle that will be restored to normal function after restoration of blood flow. An alternative nuclear medicine tracer tagged to glucose is often administered to help clarify this situation. Should the weakened heart muscle with poor blood flow demonstrate uptake and metabolism of the tagged glucose, it must be alive and will predictably regain strength with sustained blood flow restoration.

It's also important to identify the presence of nonviable tissue resulting from heart attack so that patients won't have to undergo a needless invasive revascularization procedure like stenting or coronary artery bypass grafting, because these interventions introduce additional risks (infection, clotting, stroke, heart attack) and won't restore heart function to damaged tissue. Nonviable tissue is scar tissue that can't contract the way normal heart cells do, even when blood flow is restored. Regardless of size, some infarcts are patchy, containing viable and nonviable cells, whereas others consist predominantly of nonviable tissue. PET scanning helps differentiate between these possibilities.

In individuals who have a severe coronary artery narrowing but who have not experienced a heart attack, the heart has the ability to modulate its function as a means of self-preservation. The muscle that relies on blood from the narrowed artery is completely alive but may appear weakened when a patient is at rest. PET imaging can help sort this out as well.

• • • *Fast Fact* • • •

Sleepy yet alive heart muscle, in the setting of an advanced coronary artery blockage, is termed hibernating myocardium. As the name implies, the heart muscle purposefully downregulates or reduces its vigor of contraction. This is in response to the limited availability of delivered oxygen. Once oxygen delivery is restored to normal, the pumping function also returns to normal. The mechanism for downregulation is yet to be discovered. Integral to downregulation must be the awareness of reduced tissue oxygen levels. While a hypothesis on my part, this more than likely involves a sensing and triggering mechanism at the cellular level.

• • •

Can You Still Conduct a Stress Test if I Can't Exercise?

In patients who can't exercise because of physical limitations, we simulate an exercise stress test by using a medication that generates the same responses that normally occur during exercise—increased heart rate, increased muscular contraction in heart muscle, and widening (dilation) of the coronary arteries to accommodate an increased demand for blood. This kind of testing is called pharmacological stress testing or nonexercise stress testing. It also uses echocardiography to provide information about heart function.

One agent commonly used to induce an exercise response during nonexercise stress testing is dobutamine. It's a close pharmaceutical relative of adrenaline, the hormone released by the adrenal glands. In fact, dobutamine produces the same effects as adrenaline. But it's also a very safe medication and effective for aiding heart assessment.

Administered intravenously in incremental doses at three-minute intervals, dobutamine can raise the heart rate when a patient is at rest. Although nonexercise stress testing in general won't produce the kinds of blood pressure increases that are common during exercise stress testing, the increases are significant enough for diagnostic purposes. This makes dobutamine echocardiography an effective diagnostic tool.

Dobutamine echocardiography is also effective to assess for myocardial viability (alive but sleepy heart muscle with reduced pumping capacity) after a heart attack. Should viable heart muscle be identified, revascularization in the form of stenting or bypass surgery generally will be beneficial and result in improved heart function.

How Do You Do Nuclear Imaging in a Nonexercise Stress Test?

Nonexercise pharmacological stress nuclear imaging also involves intravenous administration of pharmaceuticals to aid assessment of heart function; the most commonly used agents for nonexercise stress nuclear imaging are adenosine and Persantine (dipyridamole), both potent coronary artery vasodilators.

In a normal heart, cardiac imaging following injection with a vasodilator demonstrates uniform blood flow throughout the heart tissue. But in the presence of artery narrowing caused by atherosclerosis, the vasodilator cannot adequately exert its effect, so the imaging will reveal areas that are inadequately supplied with blood.

What Can I Do to Prevent Heart Disease?

On the whole, Americans should reduce the amount of saturated fat, trans fat, cholesterol, and total fat in their diet. It's equally important to normalize high blood pressure and high cholesterol, avoid tobacco smoke, eat a healthy diet, get regular physical activity, maintain a healthy weight, and control or delay the onset of diabetes. Taking these steps will help to significantly lower your risk of heart disease and stroke. If you still need medications to reduce your blood cholesterol, a healthy diet and active lifestyle will additionally help to lower your cholesterol and improve your overall cardiovascular health.

Chapter 6

Imaging the Heart

I maging allows cardiologists to glean important information about heart function, structure, and disease progression without opening up the chest or sliding slender instruments through the arteries. Imaging the heart is an invaluable part of the diagnostic process, and the imaging tools are growing in sophistication. In fact, it's very likely that a few years from now, medicine will use predominantly noninvasive techniques for heart imaging. But even with today's imaging tools, it's possible to produce images that rival in detail those produced by a top-grade digital camera.

The imaging tools most commonly used in cardiology include chest x-ray, transthoracic and transesophageal echocardiography, coronary angiography, intravascular ultrasound, cardiac magnetic resonance imaging, and Multislice computed tomography.

Chest X-Ray (Chest Radiography)

A chest x-ray is a test that uses a small amount of radiation to create an image of the structures within the chest, including the heart, lungs, blood vessels, and bones. Focusing a beam of radiation at

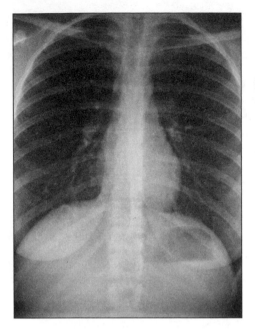

the chest produces the x-ray image. The radiation passes through the body and produces a black and white image recorded on special film or by special computer software. The resulting x-ray image looks like a giant negative from a black and white photograph. In reality, it is a compilation of shadows of varying density, depending upon the structures targeted.

X-rays record the variation in density of the body's tissues. The amount of radiation that passes through a tissue and produces a corresponding shadow on x-ray sensitive film depends on the density of that tissue. Bones, for example, are very dense, and most of the radiation can't pass through to the film. So bones appear white on an x-ray. Tissues that are less dense—such as the lungs, which are filled with air— allow more x-rays to pass through to the film, so they show up on film as shades of gray.

What Can Be Detected Using an X-Ray?

The chest x-ray is a dependable, comparatively inexpensive, and highly reliable tool for obtaining a quick view of the heart shadow and adjacent structures, and the resulting images yield valuable information. A chest x-ray can help a physician ascertain the severity of a heart condition or reveal problems that can complicate cardiac condition management. For instance, a chest x-ray can reveal or heighten suspicion for:

- Fluid in the lungs, which is a signal of congestive heart failure
- An enlarged heart shadow, which may be a sign of a prior heart attack
- Pericardial effusion, which is fluid in the pericardial sac, the thin lining around the heart
- Enlargement of a heart chamber

An x-ray can confirm the presence of atherosclerosis by revealing calcium buildup in the aorta and in the coronary arteries. It can suggest certain congenital heart defects, engorged blood vessels (a sign of pulmonary hypertension, or high blood pressure in the lungs), and aortic aneurysm, an abnormal and potentially lethal bulging defect in the vessel wall. The x-ray can also reveal an enlarged heart or be used to confirm proper placement of cardiac devices such as pacemakers or catheters (used to monitor intracardiac pressures) placed during hospitalization.

Are There Any Risks Associated with Chest X-Rays?

Chest x-rays are safe and produce no side effects. The amount of radiation produced during the procedure is very small, so the risks to adults are minimal.

· · · *Fast Fact* · · ·

A chest x-ray is a screening test devoid of the picture resolution and precision of other testing. Its greatest strengths are its widespread availability, limited cost, and low risk. It is a static picture and therefore renders no real-time assessment of heart function.

· · ·

Transthoracic Echocardiography

Transthoracic echocardiography is an external or noninvasive assessment of cardiac function. This painless method of cardiac testing produces information within minutes. It's also highly portable and, given the amount of useful information it produces, relatively inexpensive.

How Does the Echocardiogram Produce an Image of My Heart?

An echocardiogram—the image resulting from echocardiography—is produced using a device called an ultrasound transducer, 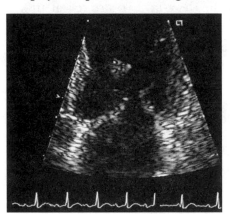 which emits high-frequency sound waves. Clear gel, which is applied to the skin of the chest, facilitates transmission of the sound waves with limited interference. The transducer, roughly similar in size and shape to a microphone, is glided over the gel. The waves painlessly penetrate skin and bone, are absorbed by the target organ—the heart, for instance—and are bounced back toward the transducer. A sophisticated computer converts the received ultrasound wave information into detailed images.

What Is Transesophageal Echocardiography?

In transesophageal echocardiography (TEE), a probe (transducer) is guided into the esophagus, the tube that leads to your stomach. Before inserting the probe, a topical anesthetic is sprayed on the throat to minimize the gag reflex; intravenous conscious sedation also is common. As the probe emits sound waves, it creates clear images of the heart and the large vessels near the heart, such as the aorta. TEE results provide information about the size of the heart and how well the valves are functioning; it can also reveal

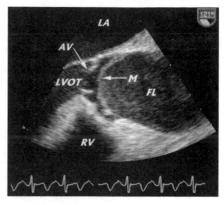

damaged heart tissue and blood clots within the heart. So TEE is a very useful tool for examining suspected cardiac and related problems as it provides clearer images compared with a surface echocardiogram, which is performed through the chest wall. Transesophageal echocardiography doesn't image through the chest wall muscles and rib cage. The images produced are obtained in real time, during actual heart motion.

What Can Be Detected Using Echocardiography?

With routine echocardiographic imaging, it's possible to assess global and regional heart problems. A global problem reflects the status of overall heart contractility; a regional problem generally involves obstruction in one of the main coronary arteries that results in localized heart muscle weakening.

Echocardiography can precisely measure cardiac chamber sizes and wall thicknesses, detect excess fluid within the pericardial space, and aid assessment of the cardiac valves. It can also identify tissue injury caused by heart attack and detect heart dysfunction in the form of myocardial scar.

After a heart attack, echocardiography is a useful follow-up test for assessing residual heart function, or for determining the presence of abnormal cardiac remodeling (abnormal enlargement of the heart) or the formation of aneurysm, an abnormal heart muscle bulge that can arise when heart attack weakens muscle tissue. (The weakened tissue bulges as it has lost its muscular contractility.)

• • • *Fast Fact* • • •

Heart attack can cause acute valvular leakage, cardiac rupture (a weakening, then tearing of the ventricle wall that results in unwanted passage of blood into the pericardial sac—an invariably fatal development), or a ventricular septal defect (hole in the muscular wall dividing the right and left ventricles). All these conditions can be identified with echocardiography. The rapidity of image acquisition is one of echocardiography's main strengths.

• • •

Thanks to the information it produces, echocardiography can guide medication therapy as to selection and dosing, and it can identify the need for electrical therapy—that is, surgical insertion of an implantable cardiac defibrillator (ICD).

Are There Any Risks Associated with Echocardiography?

Echocardiography poses no risks.

Coronary Angiography (Cardiac Catheterization or Coronary Angiogram)

Coronary angiography, which involves injecting x-ray dye to directly visualize the coronary arteries, was developed at the Cleveland Clinic in 1958 by F. Mason Sones, M.D. As is the case with many great scientific advances, it was actually by accident that Sones discovered that the heart and its arteries could be safely imaged in far greater detail and clarity than had ever before been possible. The discovery in many ways marked the beginning of modern cardiology.

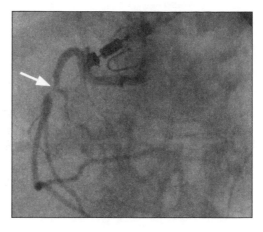

Coronary angiography is the most widely used and available tool for definitively assessing the health of the coronary arteries. Cardiologists use coronary angiography to:

- Directly visualize the coronary arteries to assess their anatomical distribution (how they're spread across the heart's surface) and to locate and determine the extent of atherosclerotic obstructions

- Measure pressures inside the heart chambers for diagnosis of valvular heart disease and to better formulate treatment options

- Evaluate heart muscle function

- Determine the need for further treatment (angioplasty/ stenting or bypass surgery)

How Is a Coronary Angiography Performed?

Coronary angiography involves inserting a catheter—a long, slender, and hollow tube—into an artery that leads to the heart. In most cases, cardiologists use the femoral artery, located in the fold between the abdomen and the upper leg, very near the groin, as the insertion point. (For many years, the common entry point for

Please Note

There are no nerves inside the blood vessels. Once the area of catheter access is anesthetized, you will not feel the catheters inside your body. The only two sensations include the doctors resting some of their equipment gently on your lap and the sensation of warmth often experienced when dye is injected into the left ventricle. The latter transpires secondary to a greater volume of dye, is not dangerous, and passes almost instantaneously.

the catheter was the brachial artery, which lies on the inside of the upper arm, at the inner elbow fold. Over time, however, interventional cardiologists determined that using the femoral artery was much less complicated and safer.)

The insertion point is first treated with a local anesthetic to minimize discomfort. Then a plastic introducer sheath (a short, hollow tube) is inserted in the artery. The introducer helps control bleeding, protects the vessel walls, and supports and guides the catheter as it's gently steered up the femoral artery via the aorta and into the coronary artery openings (ostia). As dye is injected into the heart's arteries, multiple images are recorded from many angles to provide as much complementary information as possible about the coronary artery anatomy and blood flow.

After imaging is completed, the angiography catheter is removed, and an instrument known as a pigtail catheter (so called because it is shaped similar to a pig's tail) is inserted, guided to the heart, and positioned within the left ventricle, the main pumping chamber. The pigtail catheter facilitates injection of dye into the left ventricle, permitting evaluation of diffuse and discrete heart pumping function.

What Can Be Detected Using Coronary Angiography?

Coronary angiography provides accurate information about the coronary artery blood supply to the heart and is a key source for evaluating a patient with a suspected or confirmed heart attack. It can identify or exclude—with near certainty—the presence of significant coronary artery disease. Because it produces a wealth of information about the number and pattern of artery blockages, it permits the selection of optimal therapy, whether medication only, angioplasty and stenting, or coronary artery bypass surgery.

Are There Any Risks Associated with Coronary Angiography?

Infrequent risks associated with coronary angiography include damage to the artery accessed for catheter insertion, stroke, heart attack, and death. Kidney dysfunction is also a danger because iodinated dye can be deleterious to the kidneys, especially when kidney function is already impaired. Tolerance can be determined using straightforward laboratory tests that measure kidney function.

• • • Fast Fact • • •

Coronary angiography, now available for the past 50 years, remains the definitive gold standard test to diagnose and quantify coronary artery obstructions. Despite it being the best, it suffers from the limitation of assessing a three-dimensional process—coronary atherosclerosis—utilizing two-dimensional imaging. With this inherent limitation, both over- and underestimation of coronary artery narrowing does occur. Fortunately, in experienced hands, this is an uncommon scenario.

• • •

Cardiac Magnetic Resonance Imaging (Cardiac MRI)

Cardiac magnetic resonance imaging is a noninvasive tool that produces detailed images of the heart, its vessels, and structures without the use of x-rays. Instead, cardiac MRI relies on radiofrequency waves and a large and powerful magnet to produce images. (The magnet precludes MRI use on patients with metallic implants such 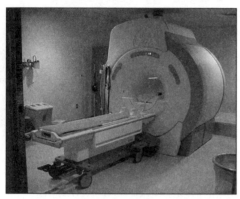 as pacemakers or implantable cardiac defibrillators; stents, however, pose no risk.)

Magnetic resonance imaging can be an alternative for patients who may have kidney dysfunction and who may not tolerate the use of iodine-based contrast agents, which are injected into the bloodstream and are required for certain cardiac imaging approaches such a CT scanning and cardiac catheterization. Computed tomography (CT scan) is similar procedurally to an MRI scan and produces detailed images noninvasively, but the CT scan relies on x-rays and, depending on the situation, injection of a contrast agent.

In certain situations, MRI is better than CT at distinguishing between tissues from different organs and body structures. Nevertheless, cardiac MRI itself may in time be displaced by a new type of CT approach called Multislice CT. MRI, unlike Multislice CT, doesn't provide high-resolution images of coronary arteries.

How Is a Cardiac MRI Performed?

Cardiac MRI imaging is performed similarly to CT imaging. An intravenous line is placed in the arm and the patient is asked to rest still on their back on the MRI table. The patient is then placed in the MRI scanner which is a large circular object containing a powerful magnet. The contrast agent gadolinium is injected into the bloodstream at the time of the test and assists with image acquisition and resolution during MRI imaging. Unlike CT imaging which takes a matter of a few minutes, MRI scanning can take 30 minutes or longer. Some patients feel claustrophobic in the MRI scanner due to its configuration coupled with the longer study length. Open MRI scanners have been developed which have lessened this concern but are not as widely available.

What Can Be Detected Using Cardiac MRI?

MRI obtains similar information to CT imaging. The two tests are complementary in the sense that CT imaging is acquired much faster and is not contraindicated should there be metal implants in the body such as a pacemaker, or hip or knee replacement. MRI does provide additive information over CT imaging and can be helpful in certain circumstances. For instance, similar to echocardiography, MRI can obtain motion pictures of your heart compared to CT imaging which produces still frames only. The cardiac motion pictures permit an assessment of heart pumping strength and also assess heart valve function. Tissue characterization of MRI is superior to CT, permitting assessment of fat and water tissue content. MRI is also the best test available to assess the pericardium, the lining of the heart.

Are There Any Risks Associated with Cardiac MRI?

Risks associated with cardiac MRI include claustrophobia (from lying inside the MRI apparatus) and skin irritation caused by the intravenous line used to administer the noniodinated contrast agent. Patients who fail to report the existence of metal objects on or inside their bodies are also at risk because of the significant magnetic field generated by the MRI. Lastly, patients with impaired kidney function may have a reaction to the gadolinium medication. It is important to have your kidney function checked via a blood test before a cardiac MRI is performed.

Multislice Computed Tomography

Multislice computed tomography (MSCT) is a comparatively new noninvasive imaging tool that can help detect "silent" heart disease earlier than traditional diagnostic tools as well as lead to a much more selective use of coronary angiography.

What Can Be Detected Using Multislice Computed Tomography?

Using a computer that quickly pieces together huge amounts of data gathered during a scan, MSCT can build detailed images of

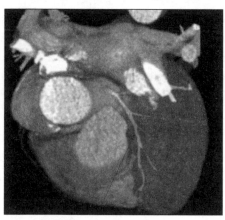

the heart's structures and vessels. The scan produces two-dimensional images that a computer program then converts into three-dimensional images with remarkable anatomic detail, which allow physicians to explore the heart from all angles. For example, MSCT can image the coronary artery wall to identify developing atherosclerosis that hasn't caused artery narrowing and that could be missed by coronary angiography given its subtlety.

Images from MSCT can also rule out the presence of atherosclerosis, detect early changes characteristic of coronary artery disease (CAD), and identify the likelihood of artery narrowing, which can later be confirmed with coronary angiography. MSCT can also provide high-resolution images somewhat comparable to those produced during intravascular ultrasound—which, as noted, is highly effective for identifying atherosclerosis; however, intravascular ultrasound is an invasive procedure. Radiation produced by MSCT approximates that of coronary angiography.

MSCT is an alternative for patients who don't want to undergo coronary angiography because of its small risks (bleeding, infection, vascular injury, and a small risk of stroke), or for patients who have atypical cardiac symptoms due to inconclusive exercise stress test results.

As the technology is refined, MSCT will potentially offer many clinical benefits:

- With patients scheduled for valve surgery, the noninvasive MSCT could be and in certain circumstances is presently used in lieu of coronary angiography to provide helpful details of heart anatomy and vessel location. Surgeons use this information to guide them during the procedure.

- For patients who have undergone a coronary artery bypass graft (CABG) procedure and who need reoperation, MSCT currently provides information to help surgeons determine the safest and most efficient way to reopen the chest without damaging the prior bypass grafts.

A current shortcoming of MSCT is "shadowing," particularly in patients who have intracoronary stents. MSCT can't reliably produce details of the area inside the stent, so it can miss restenosis (blockage in the stent), which can sometimes occur after stent placement. This is due to shadowing. Another drawback involves the heartbeat. Although MSCT is designed to capture images of the heart at rest between beats, the technology can be less effective if a patient has a heart rhythm disorder, such as atrial fibrillation.

Image acquisition and computer postprocessing is adversely affected due to the cardiac irregularity.

On the other hand, shadowing in conjunction with a decreased blood flow beyond the device can be a good indication of blockage inside the stent.

Despite its shortcomings, MSCT use is increasing and it likely will someday greatly reduce the need for diagnostic heart catheterization. Multislice technology also could be extremely helpful for assessing emergency room patients complaining of chest discomfort who don't fit the classic roster of signs associated with significant artery narrowing or heart attack. Again, this would help prevent unnecessary invasive procedures and ensure that patients who do need intervention are appropriately selected.

• • • *Fast Fact* • • •

Multislice CT as it pertains to the heart arteries is also known as CT Coronary Angiography or CTA. CTA is very good at detecting coronary artery calcification, which is a marker for coronary artery disease. At present, the image resolution for quantification of the percent of obstruction lags that of coronary angiography. As this technique is further refined, which is occurring at a rapid pace, expect to see it more prominently situated amongst our coronary artery imaging testing options.

• • •

Are There Any Risks Associated with Multislice Computed Tomography?

Risks associated with MSCT include radiation exposure and intravenous dye administration. Both are not minimal and similar in magnitude to a coronary angiogram. For this reason, there should be a dedicated discussion between you and your doctor to select the best test to image your coronary arteries. Should the MSCT demonstrate significant coronary artery blockage, a coronary angiogram will undoubtedly be recommended including additional x-ray and radiation exposure.

Intravascular Ultrasound (IVUS)

As we discussed in chapter 3, studies where IVUS was used to analyze plaque in coronary arteries led to a greatly improved understanding of coronary artery disease. IVUS is an important cardiac research tool, but it's also selectively used in daily patient care.

Like coronary angiography, IVUS involves sliding a catheter into the femoral artery and guiding it to the heart. Similar to transthoracic echocardiography, it uses ultrasound technology to produce images. But with IVUS, the imaging device is miniaturized and placed at the catheter tip.

What Can Be Detected Using Intravascular Ultrasound?

Once inside a vessel, IVUS can produce cross-sectional images that reveal even minor atherosclerosis development or narrowing that traditional imaging often overlooks. It also can be used to differentiate soft plaque from hard plaque (remember, soft plaque causes most heart attacks), and provide information that improves proper balloon and stent selection. It can be particularly helpful for monitoring heart transplant patients for development of incipient coronary artery disease, a marker of organ rejection.

Are There Any Risks Associated with Intravascular Ultrasound?

The risks of intravascular ultrasound are similar to those of coronary angiography. Unlike coronary angiography where a catheter is placed at the opening of a coronary artery, IVUS requires an ultrasound catheter in the form of a small wire to be placed inside a coronary artery. Provided this difference, there is a theoretical concern of tearing the artery or dislodging plaque. In actuality, this is not observed with any significant frequency.

Chapter 7

Medical Therapy

Medical therapy involves using medications to help prevent or manage heart disease and conditions such as high blood pressure or diabetes. Medical therapy is important because it has the potential to produce positive benefits among the largest number of patients. For example, even if patients may not have access to the most sophisticated interventions for heart disease, they can most likely obtain medicines to manage heart disease. Think of medical and interventional therapies as fishing nets: when we cast the interventional net into the waters of heart disease, we might catch—and help—10,000 patients. But when we cast the net of medical therapy into those same waters, we can help a million patients or more.

As previously discussed, primary prevention refers to using medical therapy before a cardiovascular event occurs; secondary prevention refers to medical therapy in the wake of a cardiovascular event to reduce the chances of a subsequent event.

In addition to preventing heart attack and stroke, medical therapy is used to reduce the likelihood of congestive heart failure, heart rhythm disorders, and coronary artery disease. Other benefits include decreasing high blood pressure and lowering cholesterol levels; both conditions promote the development of coronary artery disease and congestive heart failure.

Commonly used agents for preventing and managing heart disease and cardiovascular events are beta blockers, calcium channel blockers, statins, angiotensin-converting enzyme (ACE) inhibitors, and thienopyridines (for example, clopidogrel). The most commonly prescribed over-the-counter (nonprescription) agent for this purpose is aspirin. Cardiologists also may prescribe a nitrate to help manage and prevent episodes of chest pain.

How long medical therapy lasts depends on many variables. Once patients begin medicines to manage heart disease and its related conditions, they should remain under a physician's supervision. This is crucial because regular follow-up appointments are necessary to serially assess the effectiveness of medications. Perhaps dosage levels may have to be adjusted, or some medications will have to be changed altogether.

Take Alex, for example.

Alex's Story

Alex grew up in Chicago, a child of the Depression. He excelled in high school, earned an engineering degree at Cornell University, went on to the University of Pennsylvania's Wharton Business School, got married at age 32, spent two years in the military, and came back home to begin a successful career. Eventually, he went on to help run the family business, a furniture store that had been opened in 1932, shortly after Alex's father Noel lost his job. Alex's younger brother Nicholas (younger by eighteen months) followed closely behind every step of the way: high school, college, business school, the military, and later the furniture company.

When Alex and his brother Nicholas were in the military, they developed a passion for wine and good food. Both brought that passion back to the States and cultivated it throughout their lives. Neither brother ever smoked, but neither was physically active. Later in life, when Alex and Nicholas took over the family business in 1973, Alex's precious relationship with his brother changed drastically. Nicholas had his own way of doing things, and he wasn't interested in guidance from anyone about his plans or decisions. By 1997, Nicholas was living alone, estranged from his wife, estranged from his brother. On a Sunday morning in September of that year, at age 69, Nicholas dropped dead from a heart attack while he was taking a shower. (Forty-three years earlier, Noel, their father, had died from a heart attack at age 49.)

His brother's death from heart disease didn't have the effect on Alex that one might expect. It was a tremendous, tragic loss, but Nicholas had been significantly overweight, and he loved the rich food, the wine, the cognac. Was it so surprising that he went the way he did? Alex wasn't ignorant, but he did feel that he took better care of himself. He was certainly overweight, but so were a lot of men his age—in fact, his age and younger. He was never sick, and he always had energy for work.

Some years before, when he realized his brother was never going to change, Alex had sold his interest in the family business to Nicholas and set about looking for business opportunities he could get passionate about. He eventually purchased a small chain of mini-marts.

The job ended up consuming him with its constant travel from one location to the next, nurturing store managers and listening to their endless laments about finding and keeping staff while they badgered him about not having enough of this, that, or another thing. He was often away from home, and leisurely (and healthy) lunches weren't an option—he had to make the rounds. Every day he would hit a McDonald's, Burger King, Wendy's, or KFC. Alex kept up this routine five days a week—for six years. He also ate a lot of ice cream and frozen yogurt dispensed from soft-serve machines because all the mini-marts that he owned had them. It was just too easy to walk over to the machine and treat himself to a little snack.

Alex sold off the franchise in 1997, moving on to help run a specialty consulting start-up company in Cleveland; the endeavor had him flying back and forth from Chicago for a year. Sometimes during his Friday afternoon concourse sprints, he'd notice chest pain, but once he fell into his seat and got situated, the pain would dissipate. However, he knew the sensation wasn't normal, so in December of 1998 he went to see his doctor. Alex was 67 at the time. His physician didn't waste time. He said, "Alex, you need a cardiologist."

The cardiology work-up produced a diagnosis of high blood pressure and a heart catheterization demonstrated evidence of a narrowed coronary artery; however, the narrowing wasn't significant enough to warrant intervention with angioplasty or surgery. Alex was put on blood pressure medications, began taking a statin, and agreed to cut back on the wine and rich foods as well as taking up exercise to help get his weight in line. Things remained mostly stable for about six years, although given his schedule Alex found it tough to exercise or significantly modify his diet.

Alex's cardiologist had been closely monitoring his progress, and by the fall of 2005, Alex experienced recurrent chest distress. A repeat cardiac catheterization clarified that one of his arteries was getting dangerously narrow. "Alex," he said, "it's time for a stent." The procedure went smoothly, but just a few weeks afterward, still bothered by the idea of a foreign object in his body, Alex experienced chest discomfort and was convinced that the stent had moved (once deployed, stents don't move). That led him to the emergency room and more testing. The new findings showed another narrowing in a small coronary artery; Alex left the hospital with a second stent. (It's likely the narrowing was present on the first angiogram too but felt to be in a smaller artery serving less heart muscle and purposefully not instrumented at that time.)

Today, Alex has his cholesterol under much better control, and he's making progress with his weight. The stents, he says, provided almost immediate relief from heart disease symptoms. But now three variables have to be managed: blood pressure, the advancing coronary artery disease, and the stents themselves, which can become narrowed and develop clotting. Including one baby aspirin, Alex takes several medications at least once every day: hydrochlorothiazide (a diuretic and antihypertensive), atorvastatin (cholesterol-lowering agent), isosorbide dinitrate (prevents angina by reducing blood pressure and capillary pressure), atenolol (beta

Red Flag

Alex illustrates a doctor-patient conundrum. He has appropriately sought medical attention, he has undergone the requisite heart procedures, he is taking his medications, and he sees his physician for regular follow-up. His exercise and dietary habits merit significant improvement. This is an extremely common scenario. In this circumstance, I strongly recommend that Alex enroll in a formal cardiac rehabilitation program. This type of program structures an exercise schedule tailored to the individual patient in terms of ability and orthopedic limitations. It also typically incorporates didactic sessions including meeting with a dietitian, joint classes with other patients focusing on implementing and sustaining healthy heart habits, and developing a structured program once this program has concluded. These programs typically are scheduled for three times per week for six weeks, and I have found them to be extremely successful for my patients. Realizing that you have heart disease is not an easy process and requires emotional adaptation. This is greatly facilitated when you are amongst others who are working through the same sets of emotions. Collective encouragement from your peers ultimately spells success.

blocker; lowers blood pressure and heart rate), clopidogrel (blood platelet inhibitor), amlodipine (calcium channel blocker; relaxes blood vessels), ramipril (ACE inhibitor, for high blood pressure), and potassium chloride (to manage potassium deficiency).

Alex has struggled to keep his part of the heart-healthy bargain. He's 100 percent compliant about taking his medications—but exercise and diet are two different matters. He's worked hard to improve his diet: oatmeal most mornings, salad for most lunches, and dinners mostly devoid of carbs and fat. When he and his wife downsized to a condo, he invested in a treadmill, a rowing machine, even a Freestyle trainer so he could convert the condo utility room into a minifitness center. "I told my wife I'm going to start exercising. But the machines are waiting for me to get there," he admits.

Alex has been seeing his cardiologist regularly and his condition has stabilized. His cholesterol and triglyceride numbers are nearly at goal, and his blood pressure is now within the normal range. His exercise regime remains nil and his dietary choices, while slightly improved, remain haphazard as he dines out often and grabs fast food when in a pinch for time.

Aspirin

One of the most important things to remember about aspirin is that when it's used for heart disease management, it's considered a prescription medication.

Although aspirin is a nonprescription pharmaceutical, it's widely "prescribed" to patients with heart disease. In other words, regular aspirin use is considered an integral component of heart disease therapy. Interestingly, aspirin is among a select group of medications that gained over-the-counter status (it can be bought without a physician's prescription) long before the creation of what we now know as "drug testing," a process governed by the Food and Drug Administration. In fact, aspirin has been used in various forms for centuries.

It was only during the past several decades that researchers began to examine this wonder drug. Clinicians knew that aspirin would ease pain, but no one really knew how it worked. As aspirin's effects on the body were studied, two things became apparent. Besides its anti-inflammatory properties, which reduces pain severity, aspirin was found to impede the action of blood platelets, whose sole mission is to aid the blood-clotting process, and to improve blood flow in the clogged coronary artery.

In terms of aspirin's anticlotting property, keep in mind that most heart attacks result from the loss of coronary artery blood supply caused by a clot that develops at the site of unstable plaque in a narrowed vessel. When the plaque ruptures, the body reacts as if the vessel has ruptured and kicks the body's clotting and tissue repair system into action. That includes platelet activation: platelets (the "sticky" components of blood) congregate at the injury site and work with other blood products to repair the plaque rupture. In many cases, this creates a clot that severely impairs blood flow and results in heart attack.

• • • **Fast Fact** • • •

Platelets are often characterized as sticky because,
once activated, they literally stick to tissue,
each other, and additional blood components
like fibrin to form a clot.

• • •

By inactivating platelets, aspirin products impair the blood's ability to form a blood clot inside a coronary artery.

Unless a true aspirin allergy exists or if there is a history of life-threatening bleeding on aspirin, every patient with coronary artery disease should take an aspirin product daily. This is because platelets have a short life span—seven days—but the bone marrow creates new platelets daily to replace the ones that die off. Taking aspirin daily ensures that it is exerting its anticlotting effects on the greatest number of platelets. Missing a day means missing the opportunity to inactivate a new batch of platelets, and that can increase the risk of unwanted clotting.

Who Should Take Aspirin?

The American Heart Association recommends aspirin use for patients who have been diagnosed with heart attack, unstable angina, ischemic stroke (caused by a blood clot in the brain), or transient ischemic attacks (reversible neurological deficits). As stated, the main exception is the patient who is allergic to aspirin (rash, tongue swelling, severe shortness of breath) or has a medical condition that can worsen because of aspirin use. In aspirin allergic or intolerant patients, using daily clopidogrel (see page 164) instead is recommended.

Does Aspirin Have Any Side Effects?

When aspirin dosing recommendations aren't followed, it can cause side effects such as stomach pain, ulcers, excessive bruising, and internal bleeding.

Safety is the major reason to stick with a lower rather than a higher dose of aspirin. In 2002, Cleveland Clinic researchers showed that the optimal dose for daily use of aspirin is between 80 and 160 mg, or at most, half of the standard 325-mg aspirin commonly prescribed. According to this study, the lower dose is effective at inactivating platelets and reduces the risk of internal bleeding. (A baby aspirin contains 81 mg. Adult formulations in the same dosage are also available.) Patients taking Coumadin, an anticoagulant, or clopidogrel, an antiplatelet agent, should take no more than 81 mg of aspirin per day. So far, evidence doesn't suggest that a dose higher than 162 mg per day produces any more benefit than lower doses.

Since aspirin interferes with the platelet function, the most common side effect of daily aspirin use is increased ease of bruising. Even the slight bump of a wrist or hand, a common occurrence that goes unnoticed by most of us, can produce a bruise. This is particularly true in older patients, whose skin and capillaries are fragile due to age, and who already bruise easily. Thus, older persons who take aspirin are highly prone to bruising, and the prominent dark blotches that form on the skin can be quite unsettling to look at. But if a bruise doesn't bleed, there's little to worry about. In fact, bruising means that aspirin is having the intended effect on platelets.

Another possible side effect of daily aspirin use is gastrointestinal discomfort, which most often manifests as heartburn or abdominal distress.

Perhaps the biggest fear associated with aspirin use is uncontrolled bleeding in the brain, also known as hemorrhagic stroke or cerebral vascular accident (CVA). However, CVA is a rare occurrence among daily aspirin users. The cardiovascular benefit of aspirin certainly outweighs the risk of cerebrovascular bleeding in most patients.

Does Aspirin Work for Everyone?

Though it is widely available and used for a variety of purposes, aspirin is still very much a medication. Not all medications are equally effective (or safe) in every person who ingests them. Aspirin's effects on platelets can vary from person to person; in fact, it's not uncommon for aspirin to have less than a maximal platelet inhibitory effect. These patients are characterized as "aspirin resistant." This can be evaluated by a blood test and is worthwhile to discuss with your physician.

Beta Blockers

When the body is under physical or mental stress—or both—the heart rate increases to ensure adequate blood flow necessarily associated with higher oxygen demands. Stress hormones, which regulate the heart's response to stress, are released into the bloodstream by certain organs or by minuscule nerve endings situated near special sites on the surfaces of cells.

In the heart, stress hormones act on beta-1 receptors, special microscopic sites on heart muscle cells. When stimulated by the stress hormones norepinephrine and epinephrine (types of adrenaline), these beta-1 receptors signal the heart to beat harder and stronger. This action is also accompanied by the release of renin, a hormone that causes vasoconstriction (blood vessel constriction) and, in turn, an increase in blood pressure.

In a patient with an artery narrowed by atherosclerosis, an increase in the heart's workload can cause angina and labored breathing. Beta blockers—also known as beta-adrenergic blocking agents or beta-blocking agents—help prevent stress hormones from exerting their effects on beta receptors. This lightens the heart's workload by reducing the force of cardiac contraction and widens the arteries beyond the heart. The overall effect is a decrease in blood pressure, a lower resting pulse rate, and, most important, a lower heart rate during exertion or exercise. In simple terms, the heart is prevented from overtaxing itself—it needs less oxygen than it would without the beta blocker. Thus, these agents can prevent angina onset.

Research has shown that prolonged use of beta blockers can significantly reduce the likelihood of a second heart attack and help prevent development of rhythm disorders like ventricular tachycardia and fibrillation. As we discussed in chapter 3, ventricular fibrillation can cause sudden cardiac death (complete cessation of the heart's pumping action).

What Happens if I Miss a Dose When Taking a Beta Blocker?

Once a beta blocker is prescribed, it's important to adhere closely to the dosing regimen because missing a daily dose could result in rebound tachycardia (a state of abnormally fast contraction), which puts a significant amount of stress on the heart muscle and produces a greater demand for oxygen. If that demand can't be met, a person could suffer an acute heart attack or abnormal, life-threatening heart rhythms.

As previously noted, beta blockers can prevent stress hormones from exerting their effects on beta-1 receptors. When the heart is repeatedly exposed to beta blockers, the number of beta-1 receptors in heart tissue increases. This is called upregulation. Remember, when stimulated by the stress hormones norepinephrine and epinephrine, beta-1 receptors cause the heart to beat harder and stronger, and this is accompanied by an increase in blood pressure. So long as the beta blocker is present, the increase in the number of beta-1 receptors poses no problem to the patient. The drug acts on the new receptors, just as it does on the original receptors.

However, abruptly withdrawing beta blocker medication creates a whole new ball game. The increase in beta-1 receptors means there are more sites for stress hormones norepinephrine and epinephrine to act on. It's almost as if the receptors are so thirsty for the hormones, they soak them up. So if beta blocker dosing is gradually reduced over time—say, days or weeks, depending on the patient—rebound tachycardia can be avoided because the number of beta-1 receptors returns to the pre–beta blocker quantity.

Who Should Take Beta Blockers?

As is the case for aspirin, beta blockers should be prescribed to all patients who have experienced an acute heart attack unless contraindicated because of an extremely low blood pressure or pulse.

Do Beta Blockers Have Side Effects?

Side effects of beta blocker use include drowsiness, fatigue, erectile dysfunction, dizziness, worsening asthma symptoms, and dryness in the mouth, eyes, and on the skin. When side effect issues arise due to beta blocker use, the patient and physician must weigh the risks of discontinuing the medication against the incurred side effects.

The most commonly experienced beta blocker side effects are fatigue and erectile dysfunction. Both are related to the medication's ability to block the effects of norepinephrine and epinephrine. Most of the time, these side effects are tolerable; however, when fatigue or erectile dysfunction significantly impact a person's quality of life, it may be necessary to reduce the dosing levels or initiate gradual withdrawal of the medication. However, these side effects occur in the minority of circumstances.

Because beta blockers can mask the symptoms of hypoglycemia (low blood sugar), heart patients with diabetes who take these drugs have to be vigilant about eating regularly and checking blood sugar levels. This poses little difficulty except for those few diabetics with extremely labile (unpredictable high and low) blood sugar levels.

Statins

Cholesterol-lowering agents known as statins have been used since 1987 to manage high cholesterol levels. They're among the best-known and most effective medications in the heart medicine arsenal. Even more crucial, statins help stabilize plaque that's prone to rupture, and they slow the progression of atherosclerosis in arteries inside and outside the heart. All of this helps reduce the chances of heart attacks and strokes. Bottom line—statins save lives!

Diet and exercise are the safest nonpharmacological strategies for lowering cholesterol levels, but there are a number of reasons—

heredity, diabetes, socioeconomic status, physical limitations, a lack of time, family responsibilities, and discipline—that prevent people from losing weight and working out. Also, to cut the risk of experiencing a first or subsequent cardiovascular event, sometimes patients need to get cholesterol levels under control faster than can be achieved with diet and exercise alone.

Any medication that can quickly, safely, and significantly lower cholesterol levels, as well as reduce heart attack and death rates remains an asset to cardiovascular disease management. Now, this doesn't mean that anyone taking a statin is absolved from exercise or eating a healthy diet, managing diabetes, quitting smoking, or losing weight. What it means is that when prescribed under the auspices of a physician, statins can help keep cholesterol levels at their optimal levels, particularly if you exercise regularly and maintain a healthy diet. Think of it this way: statin therapy for heart disease is a 50-50 proposition, with the physician and the medications, including a statin, making up half of the deal, and the patient's vigilance and discipline as the other half. Patients who want to control their cholesterol must hold up their end of the deal.

The technical name for a statin is HMG-CoA reductase inhibitor. The name derives from the statin's ability to block HMG-CoA reductase, a liver enzyme that plays a key role in cholesterol synthesis in the liver. Although cholesterol is normally ingested in the diet, the liver produces about 85 percent of the cholesterol found in the body. The liver does this because the body needs cholesterol; cells can't function without it. The problem is that too much cholesterol isn't helpful because excess cholesterol travels the bloodstream, and over time, small amounts of it lodge within the underlayers of artery walls. This can occur in any artery, but it's particularly problematic in coronary arteries. It is believed that cholesterol may gain access to this underlayer through tiny tears in the endothelium, the smooth, very thin inner artery lining that's in constant contact with blood.

It's not exactly clear what causes the initial injury to the endothelium, but we know the most common and problematic sites of occurrence: the aorta, the carotid arteries, and the coronary arteries. Unless steps are taken to halt or diminish atherosclerosis development, what starts out as a microscopic pile of debris can evolve into a major land mass with volcanic tendencies that result in heart attack.

• • • Fast Fact • • •

It's interesting that often the most severe blockages occur at major branch points. Researchers have postulated that these branch points produce heightened blood flow turbulence and blood flow velocities, placing increased stress on and possibly disrupting the endothelial layer of the coronary arterial vessel.

• • •

What Do Lipids Have to Do with Cholesterol?

Although just about everyone knows about cholesterol, people are less familiar with the word *lipid.* But a discussion of coronary artery disease is really a discussion about lipids, which are commonly called blood fats. Lipids are fatty, waxy substances in the bloodstream that various body systems use for energy. The main components of the blood fats are triglycerides, high-density lipoproteins, low-density lipoproteins, and cholesterol.

High- and low-density lipoproteins are the good and bad cholesterols, respectively—although, as you might imagine, it's a bit more complicated than simply good versus bad. Lipoproteins ferry cholesterol throughout the body, and it's the nefarious low-density lipoprotein that's apparently responsible for damage to artery walls.

High-density lipoproteins, on the other hand, are believed to help pull that bad cholesterol from the atherosclerotic dumps and send it on its way out of the body, via the liver.

• • • *Fast Fact* • • •

A lipid panel is a blood test used to provide valuable information about blood fat levels and certain blood/ fat ratios. A lipid panel measures levels of total cholesterol, triglycerides, HDL and LDL, and very-low-density lipoprotein, and calculates the ratios of total cholesterol to HDL and LDL to HDL. The lipid panel is the starting point for cholesterol management.

• • •

How Do Statins Affect Good Cholesterol and Bad Cholesterol?

Statins can modestly raise HDL levels, an important achievement in atherosclerosis management because it's believed HDL helps pull LDL cholesterol out of artery walls so that both can be excreted altogether. Statins are also believed to lower levels of utra sensative C-reactive protein and thus lessen the degree of arterial inflammation associated with atherosclerosis.

The main effect of a statin, however, is to lower the levels of circulating LDL cholesterol. This is important because research performed at the Cleveland Clinic and elsewhere has repeatedly demonstrated that lowering LDL cholesterol levels reduces heart attack incidence.

The National Cholesterol Education Program. The evidence regarding the association between high LDL levels and cardiovascular events is so strong that LDL is considered a major marker for

Adult Treatment Panel III Classification of Total, LDL, and HDL Cholesterol (mg/dL)*

Total cholesterol	Classification
<200	Desirable
200–239	Borderline high
>240	High

LDL cholesterol	Classification
<100	Optimal
100–129	Near optimal/above optimal
130–159	Borderline high
160–189	High
>190	Very high

HDL cholesterol	Classification
<40	Low
40-59	Intermediate
>60	High (for HDL, "high" is good)

LDL = low-density lipoprotein; HDL = high-density lipoprotein; mg/dL = milligrams per deciliter (cholesterol levels are measured in milligrams per deciliter of blood)

* "Third Report of the Expert Panel on Detection, Evaluation, and Treatment of High Blood Cholesterol in Adults (Adult Treatment Panel III): Executive Summary," National Cholesterol Education Program; National Heart, Lung, and Blood Institute; National Institutes of Health. NIH Publication No. 01-3670, May 2001, and "High Blood Cholesterol: What You Need to Know," National Cholesterol Education Program; National Heart, Lung, and Blood Institute; National Institutes of Health. NIH Publication No. 05-3290, revised June 2005.

heart attack risk, and LDL is now a major target of heart disease management. This association also caused the National Cholesterol Education Program (NCEP) Expert Panel on Detection, Evaluation, and Treatment of High Blood Cholesterol in Adults in 2001 to revise its recommendations regarding LDL levels, from 130 to 100 mg/dL for high-risk patients. This significantly broadened the number of candidates who stood to benefit from statin therapy.

Then in 2004, with new data from five different studies examining statins, the NCEP refined its 2001 recommendations because these studies provided new information about different groups that used statins, such as older persons and those at very high risk for a heart attack. The current recommendations for cholesterol levels is shown on page 99.

According to NCEP, for individuals considered "very high risk" for heart disease or heart attack, an optimal LDL target is less than 70 mg/dL. For example, you'd be considered very high risk if you already have coronary artery disease and multiple cardiovascular disease risk factors, including diabetes and smoking, or you have high triglyceride levels and low HDL levels.

The revised NCEP cholesterol guidelines also outline recommendations for high-cholesterol treatment, based on a formula that puts patients into four risk groups:[*]

- **Category I, Highest Risk:** Your LDL goal is less than 100 mg/dL. You need to begin the therapeutic lifestyle changes (TLC) diet to reduce your high risk even if your LDL is below 100 mg/dL. (TLC includes a cholesterol-lowering diet, physical activity, and weight management.) You may also need to start the TLC diet and drug treatment with a cholesterol-lowering agent (a statin) if you have had a recent heart attack or have heart disease and diabetes. Medication treatment is also recommended if your LDL is 100 mg/dL or above.

---

[*] "High Blood Cholesterol: What You Need to Know," National Cholesterol Education Program; National Heart, Lung, and Blood Institute; National Institutes of Health. NIH Publication No. 05-3290, revised June 2005.

- **Category II, High Risk:** Your LDL goal is less than 130 mg/dL. If your LDL is 130 mg/dL or above, you need to begin treatment with the TLC diet. If your LDL is still 130 mg/dL or more after three months on the TLC diet, a cholesterol-lowering agent along with the TLC diet is recommended. If your LDL is less than 130 mg/dL, you need to follow the heart-healthy diet designated for all Americans, which allows a little more saturated fat and cholesterol than the TLC diet does.

- **Category III, Moderate Risk:** Your LDL goal is less than 130 mg/dL. If your LDL is 130 mg/dL or above, you need to begin the TLC diet. If your LDL is 160 mg/dL or more after three months on the TLC diet, a cholesterol-lowering agent along with the TLC diet is recommended. If your LDL is less than 130 mg/dL, you will need to follow the heart-healthy diet designated for all Americans.

- **Category IV, Low-to-Moderate Risk:** Your LDL goal is less than 160 mg/dL. If your LDL is 160 mg/dL or above, you need to begin the TLC diet. If your LDL is 160 mg/dL or more after three months on the TLC diet, a cholesterol-lowering agent along with the TLC diet is recommended, especially if your LDL is 190 mg/dL or more. If your LDL is less than 160 mg/dL, you will need to follow the heart-healthy diet.

You can learn more about the NCEP cholesterol guidelines by visiting the National Heart, Lung, and Blood Institute website (*http://www.nhlbi.nih.gov*). To learn about the TLC diet, visit the American Heart Association website at *www.americanheart.org*. For the diet recommended for patients with serious heart disease, see Appendix 2 on page 211.

It's worth adding here that everyone—even people whose family history, cholesterol levels, and risk factor profiles present an outstanding picture of health and low likelihood of heart disease—should be on the therapeutic lifestyle change diet recommended by NCEP. Why? Because the most effective heart disease management program involves prevention of the development of atherosclerosis and its associated complications (heart attack and stroke). For the record, it's never too early to begin this proactive program. Additionally, there's no good reason not to introduce and maintain a healthy diet for children.

Who Should Take Statins?

The current practice is to place all patients diagnosed with arterial vascular disease on a statin, regardless of their lipid values. The reason, as previously mentioned, is that statins not only lower levels of blood lipids and modestly raise HDL levels, they also help stabilize plaque. Reducing the incidence of plaque rupture will also decrease the incidence of stroke and heart attack. Statins, then, can help prevent death from cardiovascular disease. When a statin is prescribed to a patient with arterial vascular disease, the main lipid target is LDL cholesterol. Although the recommended goal is an LDL value less than or equal to 100 mg/dL, many physicians shoot for the more aggressive LDL target of less than or equal to 70 mg/dL. Along with beta blockers and aspirin, statins have significantly improved the ability to manage cardiovascular disease, and the number of prescriptions written for these cholesterol-lowering agents will continue to rise.

Do Statins Have Side Effects?

In general, statins are overwhelmingly safe drugs; a very small percentage of patients who use them may develop side effects that warrant altering statin dosing. Among patients who adversely react to statins, the most common physical developments are muscle achiness, cramping, weakness, or tenderness; the most common physiological development is liver damage, which is characterized by reversible increases in the liver enzymes alanine aminotransferase and aspartate aminotransferase (ALT and AST). A third possible statin complication is rhabdomyolysis, which involves the breakdown of the muscle fiber myoglobin and release of it into the bloodstream; although quite serious, this side effect is extremely rare.

Muscle symptoms associated with statin use can be a sign of myalgia or myositis. Although myalgia and myositis share symptoms—achiness, cramping, and tenderness—myositis is also characterized by damage and inflammation to muscle tissue. The only way to "see" this damage is with a blood test that measures levels of the enzyme creatine phosphokinase (CPK). Muscle cells that are injured or inflamed release CPK.

In most cases, blood testing from myalgia patients shows normal CPK levels; in myositis patients, CPK levels are elevated. In both cases, the problem can be resolved by reducing statin dosing, quitting the statin, or switching to another statin because patients may react differently to different statins. It should be emphasized that myositis is a rare consequence of statin administration.

If a patient's CPK enzymes are elevated, statin dosage is reduced. But if CPK levels are very high—at least three times higher than normal—statin use is stopped to avoid permanent damage to muscle tissue and to the kidneys (caused by the increased blood load of CPK). Less than 5 percent of all patients taking statins will develop myositis.

Most patients who develop muscle cramping—it typically arises a week or two after starting on a statin—don't have myositis. But even when no clinical evidence of myositis is present, fear about the condition may cause patients to quit the statin or use it irregularly if the cramping persists. This reduces the statin's beneficial effects. Cramping can be managed by reducing the dosage or prescribing it every other day, as opposed to daily. Instead of stopping the medication on your own, consult your physician.

All patients prescribed a statin should be thoroughly educated about the difference between muscle cramping that poses no danger and the more sinister muscle inflammation. Because of potential damage to the muscles and liver, all patients who are prescribed statins should undergo regular follow-up with a physician, and these office visits should include testing to monitor blood levels of CPK, AST, and ALT. Proper statin monitoring involves blood and liver function testing three months after a patient starts the drug (or three months after a dose is increased or decreased) and, if things look satisfactory, every six months thereafter.

Liver enzyme elevation is very manageable by simply stopping statin use, at which point the situation will resolve within months without any residual organ damage. If myositis and liver abnormalities aren't an issue, but cramping is, the physician and patient should work diligently to identify an acceptable dosing regimen as statins play a key role in helping prevent heart attacks—by as much as 20 percent—by helping tame atherosclerosis and inflammation, and by stabilizing unstable plaque, the heart attack catalyst. In short, statins are believed to reduce the vigor of the atherosclerotic inflammatory process. It's safe to assume that all patients taking a statin derive protection from cardiovascular events, particularly high-risk patients and those with documented coronary artery disease (with or without a heart attack).

What Are Some of the Most Commonly Prescribed Statins?

Some commonly prescribed statins are:

- Atorvastatin (LIPITOR)
- Fluvastatin (Lescol)
- Lovastatin (MEVACOR)

- Pravastatin (Pravachol)
- Simvastatin (ZOCOR)
- Rosuvastatin (CRESTOR)

• • • *Fast Fact* • • •

Despite the demonstrated overwhelming benefits
of statins, they remain underprescribed both in number
and dosage. The potential benefit of a statin in
a patient diagnosed with coronary artery disease
dwarfs the likelihood of a potential side effect. As long
as scheduled follow-up with your physician including
regularly scheduled blood testing is maintained, the
likelihood of developing serious irreversible liver or
muscle damage from statins is low.

• • •

ACE Inhibitors

All patients who have a history of heart attack and heart muscle weakening (left ventricular systolic dysfunction) should be on an angiotensin-converting enzyme inhibitor (ACE inhibitor) and a beta blocker unless contraindicated.

The ACE inhibitor was originally developed as a medication for managing high blood pressure. This class of medication interferes with the renin-angiotensin system, which uses the hormone renin to help regulate blood pressure and blood volume by controlling the arterial smooth muscle "tone." Higher renin and angiotensin levels cause tightening and narrowing of the vessel (vasoconstriction), which increases blood pressure and raises resistance to blood pumped out of the heart. By blocking the renin-angiotensin system, the ACE inhibitor causes widening of the arteries (vasodilation) which, in turn, lowers blood pressure and reduces vessel resistance to heart output and blood flow. If ACE inhibitors had a motto, it would be "Just let the blood flow."

Who Should Take ACE Inhibitors?

The ACE inhibitor's effect is beneficial for patients whose heart has been damaged, thus weakened, by a heart attack. With ACE inhibitor administration, resistance to heart pumping is reduced, and blood flow and oxygenation of the tissues are improved. Also, by reducing the heart's workload, an ACE inhibitor can reduce the likelihood of thickening of the ventricular walls (hypertrophy). It can also reduce the likelihood of adverse heart remodeling, such as the development of a heart aneurysm. This means that patients taking an ACE inhibitor are less likely to develop heart failure; if it does develop, it tends to be less severe than in patients who have not been administered an ACE inhibitor. ACE inhibitors can also reduce the likelihood of a second heart attack.

But the most significant benefits associated with ACE inhibitor use come in the form of prevention of vascular events such as stroke and heart attack and their related conditions. The study that revealed these incredible findings tested the ACE inhibitor ramipril in people with evidence of heart disease or diabetes. These were prime candidates for heart attack and stroke. Ramipril reduced the rates of death, heart attack, stroke, and heart failure in a significant number of high-risk patients. These are patients who also typically suffer from or develop diabetes. The study also showed that ramipril could help reduce the number of complications associated with diabetes and reduce the number of new diabetes cases. A similar study conducted in Europe, using the ACE inhibitor perindopril, produced similar findings. We don't know why the ACE inhibitor offers these diabetic and vascular benefits, but the fact that it does makes it an important weapon in the fight against vascular disease events.

Do ACE Inhibitors Have Side Effects?

ACE inhibitors are very tolerable medications, but they can cause a side effect that's more annoying than problematic: chronic cough. Some patients taking an ACE inhibitor develop a persistent dry nuisance cough that's so disruptive to their quality of life, they quit the medication. It will stop shortly after the medication is discontinued. Fortunately, this transpires in only a small percentage of those patients administered an ACE inhibitor.

The improved blood flow associated with ACE inhibitor use is usually beneficial throughout the body—but in the kidneys, for instance, the decrease in blood pressure can undermine function, slowing the filtering ("cleaning") of blood and the ongoing elimination of waste products. In rare cases, ACE inhibitors can affect normal kidney function (characterized by increases in blood urea nitrogen and potassium), but vigilant monitoring and blood testing—two weeks after a patient begins taking the medication and every six months thereafter—minimize the chances of such a problem progressing without having to stop the medication. Similar to the nuisance dry cough, kidney dysfunction with ACE inhibitor administration is an uncommon occurrence and does not preclude prescribing the medication. The importance is maintaining close follow-up with your physician including follow-up blood testing.

Calcium Channel Blockers

Like ACE inhibitors, calcium channel blockers are vasodilators that help relax the blood vessels to lower blood pressure. By helping minimize passage of calcium into heart muscle cells and the smooth muscle cells of arteries (cells use calcium for contraction), calcium channel blockers relax heart muscle tissue and dilate arteries throughout the body. This helps lower blood pressure and heart rate, reduces the pumping burden on the heart, and improves blood flow to the heart.

Calcium blockers also slow the heart's electrical (conduction) system, which results in lower heart rates whether one is resting or engaging in physical activity.

Who Should Take Calcium Channel Blockers?

Calcium channel blockers are effective medicines for managing angina because they help decrease the force of heart contraction and exercise-attained heart rate, therefore reducing cardiac workload.

The vasodilating effects of calcium channel blockers work best on healthy arteries, not on those already narrowed by atherosclerosis. In fact, this is a pitfall of the calcium channel blocker. Improved blood flow in healthy coronary arteries exceeds the improvement attained in those with atherosclerosis, creating the adverse and unwanted phenomenon of "coronary artery steal"— where blood from a healthy artery "steals" or reroutes blood otherwise traveling to a nearby diseased coronary artery. In such cases, the calcium channel blocker makes a bad situation worse. Because of this drawback, calcium blockers are not used as first-line agents for coronary artery disease management. Instead, they are prescribed for patients who are already on beta blockers and nitrates (nitroglycerin preparations) but who experience persistent angina symptoms.

Unlike beta blockers, calcium channel blockers haven't been shown to reduce the incidence of heart attacks or extend life in people with heart disease; in fact, some study results have shown that patients with coronary artery disease taking calcium channel blockers fare worse than those who don't take these drugs.

Two drugs in the calcium channel blocker subclass, however, are exceptions: amlodipine and felodipine. These agents are called dihydropyridine calcium blockers and are very effective for high blood pressure management; they're also beneficial for patients who suffer from coronary artery vasospasm, a spasm that briefly narrows a coronary artery and impedes blood flow to heart tissue, thus causing angina. In such cases, combining a dihydropyridine calcium blocker with a nitrate is a very effective means of managing coronary artery vasospasm and its symptoms.

Do Calcium Channel Blockers Have Side Effects?

Since calcium channel blockers lower blood pressure and heart rate, fatigue is possible. Lightheadedness or near fainting can occur in extreme circumstances, such as overdosage, when the heart rate and/or blood pressure is severely lowered. Constipation can be problematic, particularly with the calcium channel blockers verapamil and diltiazem, but does not typically require discontinuing the medication.

Warfarin

Warfarin is an additional medication with anticlotting properties possessing a role in managing heart disease. Warfarin is better known by the brand name Coumadin.

In patients with obstructive coronary artery disease, warfarin does not reduce heart attack risk. In patients who have undergone bypass surgery, there's no evidence that warfarin helps maintain adequate blood flow in the new graft or reduces heart attack risk or death.

Who Should Take Warfarin?

Warfarin's anticlotting properties are beneficial for patients whose heart attack results in a left ventricular thrombus, a life-threatening blood clot in the heart's left ventricle. These clots are most often identified by echocardiography or angiography.

Warfarin is also prescribed to patients who suffer from recurrent heart rhythm disorders in the heart's upper chambers, such as atrial flutter or atrial fibrillation, who are at increased risk for blood clot formation within the heart. This is particularly true in patients 65 years and older, or in patients 65 years and under who have known structural heart disease (prior heart attack, valve disease, weakened heart muscle, etc.). Another group of patients in which warfarin is essential includes those with mechanical (metallic) heart valves.

Does Warfarin Have Side Effects?

The side effects of warfarin include the potential for easy bruising and bleeding. This is particularly true when warfarin is necessarily administered with aspirin or clopidogrel. To ensure the correct dosage of warfarin, a periodic blood test is warranted. This test, called an INR value, measures in seconds the degree of blood thinning. For most patients, a goal INR value is between 2.0 and 3.0 seconds. If the INR value returns significantly higher than 3.0 seconds, bleeding is more likely. If the INR value is less than 2.0 seconds, the benefit derived from taking warfarin is diminished. Warfarin also interacts with many different medications. For instance, a multitude of antibiotics potentiate (enhance) the effect of warfarin, causing unexpectedly high INR values. For this reason, it is exceedingly important that you communicate to any new healthcare provider that you are taking warfarin should a new prescription medication be contemplated. In addition, over-the-counter and herbal medications may also impact warfarin's blood thinning ability and should not be ingested while taking warfarin medication.

Thienopyridines

The currently available thienopyridine most commonly used in cardiac patients is clopidogrel, known by the brand name Plavix.

Studies testing clopidogrel in patients with stable coronary artery disease have not shown it to be more effective at interfering with platelet activity than aspirin; nor has it been shown to reduce the rate of heart attack or death. In fact, when taken in conjunction with aspirin, it was recently found to increase the bleeding ratio.

Who Should Take Clopidogrel?

Clopidogrel is useful as a substitute for aspirin in aspirin-resistant and aspirin-allergic patients.

Research has demonstrated that clopidogrel can be used after coronary artery stent implantation. For patients who receive coated or drug-eluting stents (a medicine-coated stent), taking clopidogrel for a minimum of twelve months without interruption after implantation reduces the likelihood of clot formation inside the stent. For noncoated or bare metal stents, it is currently recommended to take clopidogrel for a minimum of three months without interruption after implantation. The exact duration of optimal clopidogrel administration after intracoronary stent implantation is unknown. Current practice is to continue clopidogrel for a minimum of twelve months and often longer should no bleeding complications ensue. This is exceedingly important to prevent blood clot formation within a stent, termed stent thrombosis. Stent thrombosis can be sudden, abruptly occlude a coronary artery, and cause heart attack and death without warning.

Does Clopidogrel Have Side Effects?

Similar to warfarin, clopidogrel can result in excessive bruising and bleeding. Unlike warfarin and similar to aspirin, no blood tests are warranted to follow blood levels and to assess the effectiveness of blood thinning. There are no significant medication interactions with clopidogrel.

Nitrates

Nitrates relax the blood vessels, allowing more blood to deliver oxygen to the body's cells, including heart muscle cells. Nitroglycerin, the most commonly prescribed nitrate, is available in several forms, including tablets that are placed under the tongue (sublingual), placed between the cheek and gum (buccal), controlled-release (long-acting) tablets that are ingested, a patch, and an oral spray.

Nitroglycerin sublingual tablets and nitroglycerin spray are used to relieve discomfort during angina attacks. Long-acting nitrate preparations reduce and may prevent angina from arising during activities known to provoke attacks, like climbing stairs, sexual activity, walking uphill, and being outside in cold weather.

Who Should Take Nitroglycerin?

Nitroglycerin is most often prescribed to patients who suffer from angina pectoris despite optimal coronary artery revascularization in the form of angioplasty, stenting, or coronary artery bypass grafting. You might ask why you might experience cardiac chest discomfort after undergoing a revascularization procedure. While the advances in coronary artery revascularization are immense, small arteries, arteries with multiple blockages in a row, and arteries with complete occlusions can produce ongoing chest discomfort, improved with nitroglycerin administration. Nitroglycerin preparations improve quality of life, but no studies have demonstrated a reduction in heart attack or death rates.

Do Nitrates Have Side Effects?

The main risk associated with nitrates is the onset of low blood pressure (hypotension). In rare circumstances, this can cause significant lightheadedness or fainting. Sudden, significant blood pressure lowering can also interfere with adequate blood flow to the brain, which could potentially result in a stroke.

Repetitive, frequent use of nitrates, or use that exceeds the recommended prescribed frequency, can result in medication tolerance (tachyphylaxis). In fact, nitrates commonly lose their effectiveness if they're administered too frequently or for prolonged periods at regular intervals.

In summary, physicians have at their disposal a full complement of outstanding medications. When these medications are administered to patients with obstructive coronary artery disease, they have been demonstrated to confer significant benefit in terms of heart attack prevention and reduced death rates. The coronary artery disease patient, especially those patients who have experienced a myocardial infarction, can expect to be prescribed daily medications in the form of aspirin, a beta blocker, a statin, an ace inhibitor, and possibly clopidogrel depending if an intracoronary stent was placed. All of these medications have been closely studied in carefully conducted scientific studies with uniform agreement amongst healthcare professionals supporting their administration.

Chapter 8

Intervention

W hen an artery becomes so narrowed or clogged that its blood flow resembles a slow-leaking faucet, and the tissue that relies on blood from that vessel is at risk of dying from oxygen starvation, it's time to intervene.

The blood flow needs to be restored either by widening the artery or by finding a way to reroute the blood around the blocked artery. Widening the artery and then propping it open with a stent is performed by interventional cardiologists. Rerouting the blood flow involves implanting a new blood vessel that will take over the workload for the obstructed coronary artery. This open-chest operation is called coronary artery bypass graft surgery (CABG) or, more commonly, bypass surgery, and it's performed by cardio-thoracic surgeons.

So, how do we decide who gets what? That's not an easy question to answer because there are many variables to consider: the patient's age, health status, whether the narrowing is being diagnosed for the first time, which coronary arteries are involved, the extent of the atherosclerosis inside those arteries, and the resources and expertise of the heart center managing the case.

Bypass can be hard on the body, and recuperation can last weeks or months. So it generally favors people who are fairly fit and devoid of significant additional illnesses. Widening an artery with angioplasty and propping it open with a stent can be done without surgically opening up the chest, so there's minimal need for hospitalization, plus recuperation is fast—just a few days or more. Patients who in the past would have routinely undergone bypass surgery now receive multiple stents, with good results.

Both procedures improve blood flow and reduce the likelihood of chest discomfort resulting from exertion. But with either procedure, there's no guarantee that new narrowing or clogging won't happen. Plenty of patients undergo angioplasty and do fine for years before needing more intervention. The same is true for bypass patients. How well a patient fares after the intervention depends on the patient.

Heart attack patients who continue to experience angina or display evidence of viable heart cells within the infarct (heart attack) zone are at higher risk for another heart attack. These patients almost uniformly undergo cardiac catheterization with the intent of restoring adequate blood flow, either by angioplasty and stenting or CABG.

Some patients are better suited for CABG than others. Risk factors associated with the procedure include advanced patient age, long-standing diabetes with complications including renal insufficiency (kidney dysfunction), severe vascular disease including cerebral vascular disease and prior stroke, and reduced cognitive abilities that may negatively affect recovery from open-heart surgery. That being said, open-heart surgery has proved over the years to be an extremely safe procedure with mortality at experienced medical centers at approximately 5 percent or less.

Stents

Previously, patients with multiple advanced coronary artery blockages—several arteries with single blockages, or one or more arteries with multiple blockages—were recommended for CABG. This was particularly common for patients with a severe narrowing in the left main coronary artery and multiple vessel blockages with abnormal heart function (reduced left ventricular systolic function). Intervention with multiple stents in these patients was considered too risky because of the high likelihood of renarrowing (restenosis) at the stent sites; plus, the research data supported CABG.

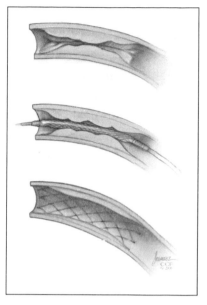

Advances in stenting technique and stent design mean more patients can safely benefit from the implantation of these devices. For instance, drug-eluting stents, which gradually release an embedded medication from the stent surface, assist in reducing the incidence of renarrowing and the need for repeat angioplasty and stent deployment within a previously placed stent. As stent technology continues to advance, an increasing number of patients who in the past would have been managed with bypass surgery can now be managed with stents, even if this involves multiple stent implantations in several coronary arteries.

• • • *Fast Fact* • • •

Despite the advances and witnessed successes of intracoronary stent placement, CABG remains a preferred option for some patients. It is important to remember that stents have been available for a period of years whereas CABG has been available and studied for decades. CABG has outstanding longitudinal data supporting its positive impact on quality of life and life extension.

• • •

Angioplasty and Stenting

Balloon angioplasty has been in use since the 1980s to help widen narrowed arteries. Cardiologists know the procedure as percutaneous transluminal coronary angioplasty (PTCA): *percutaneous,* for performed through the skin; *transluminal,* for passing a catheter through the lumen of blood vessels; *coronary,* for heart artery; and *angioplasty,* for procedural repair of a blood vessel. Angioplasty is just one of many catheter-based procedures used to examine, image, and repair the heart. Catheter-based procedures are among the techniques used in interventional cardiology.

Is Angioplasty a Risky Procedure?

PCTA is considered a less invasive technique for gaining access to the heart because there's no need to open the chest surgically. "Less

Some Limitations of Intervention

Some patients diagnosed with coronary artery disease should not undergo angioplasty and stenting or bypass surgery. In patients who've experienced heart attack, the damage caused to the tissue downstream from the obstruction is sometimes so extensive that revascularization won't produce much benefit. The blood supply can be increased to the damaged area, but because the tissue is nonviable (100 percent scarred), the increased blood flow won't improve heart function. Intervention in such cases only exposes the patient to unnecessary risks. If the tissue is viable, angioplasty and stenting or CABG, depending on the number and location of the blockages, are warranted to help improve the patient's heart health. We can make such determinations about the extent of tissue damage using an array of previously described cardiac imaging tests.

invasive" should never be equated with "no risk." Besides, PCTA is invasive, in that an artery is carefully punctured and used as a conduit to slip instruments into the body.

Catheterization involves sliding a slender and pliant tube (the catheter) into part of an artery situated either near the groin or at the inside of the upper arm near the elbow fold. This is the entry point for a host of willowy instruments that will be carefully guided through vessels leading to the heart, using low-dose x-ray as the roadmap. In angioplasty, a balloon-tipped wire is snaked through the vessels leading to a narrowed heart artery. At the site of the narrowing, the balloon is inflated; this action helps compress bulging plaque against the arterial wall to improve blood flow through a narrowed opening (lumen).

How Do Angioplasty and Stenting Work Together?

After stents were approved for use in 1994, PCTA increasingly became a two-part procedure: widening with balloon angioplasty, then stent placement to prop open the artery. When used in combination with stenting, angioplasty is referred to as pre dilation of the atherosclerotic plaque. Stenting is preferred because approximately one-third of coronary arteries undergo renarrowing after angioplasty. Also, although it occurs rarely, an artery wall can collapse after balloon angioplasty, and this can be a life-threatening event requiring emergency bypass surgery. So the stent helps ensure adequate blood flow in the artery with a lessened restenosis rate, plus it significantly reduces the risk of vessel collapse.

Angioplasty and stenting also involve x-ray imaging and dye injection, which allow the interventional cardiologist to ensure that the balloon is properly situated prior to inflation, that the artery is adequately widened after deflation, and that the stent is properly placed before being locked in place (deployed).

Several months after stenting, most patients undergo stress testing to ensure that the stent is doing its job and that the artery has not renarrowed.

Stents and Restenosis. Stents come in many lengths and diameters. One key to successful stent placement is choosing the correct size stent for a narrowed vessel section; another is ensuring that the stent is fully expanded at the target site inside the artery. Stent size is determined by the interventional cardiologist, who uses various calculations based on imaging data obtained during coronary angiography.

Although stents were designed to prevent artery narrowing after angioplasty, stent placement can breed obstruction problems. Scar tissue can and does develop around the stent surface, resulting in an obstruction that requires intervention, typically involving a redo angioplasty. This occurs about 25 percent of the time. Now that we're using drug-coated (drug-eluting) stents, this frequency is now about 10 percent. This is a significant advance!

During the first few months after a stent is placed, cells that form the artery lining (the endothelium) begin growing on and around the stent surface, almost like an extremely thin covering of wet moss. This is actually a good thing, because it makes clot formation inside the stent less likely as time passes. But placing a stent also causes fine damage to the artery wall, and as that damage heals, smooth muscle cells build up, and scar tissue forms around stent surfaces. This is a serious, certainly unwanted development because it means that renarrowing, or restenosis, is occurring. Restenosis arising from artery wall injury occurs in both women and men and is particularly a problem in people with diabetes. Restenosis can occur in anyone who gets a stent.

If restenosis occurs at the stent site, it does so mostly within the first few months of placement. You should also understand an important distinction: restenosis is not atherosclerosis. In restenosis, the culprit is the rapid smooth muscle cell accumulation that essentially forms scar tissue; in slowly developing atherosclerosis, the culprit is cholesterol and other biologic debris. Restenosis typically develops much faster than atherosclerosis, within a period of weeks to months.

Drug-eluting stents help slow the proliferation of smooth muscle cells. So far, there is no evidence of significant side effects associated with drug-eluting stents, and they have been used to good effect in patients to reduce restenosis rates.

• • • *Fast Fact* • • •

One type of stent is actually embedded with a chemotherapeutic agent. This medication is extremely low dose and delivered locally via a slow release mechanism to the stented vessel with the intent of mitigating the smooth muscle reparative response to local tissue injury following stent deployment.

• • •

Clot Management. One way to reduce the likelihood of clot formation is to administer antiplatelet medications, which interfere with the clotting process. Several different anticlotting agents—aspirin, clopidogrel, and abciximab—are used to help manage clotting associated with angioplasty and stenting. During the procedure itself, abciximab is typically administered intravenously; aspirin and clopidogrel are taken orally.

Clopidogrel is taken before and after the procedure; in fact, it should be taken religiously every day for at least nine to twelve months following the intervention. It's during this time that a patient is at highest risk for stent-associated acute blood clot formation (thrombosis). Many cardiologists encourage patients to remain on clopidogrel for at least one year to minimize the chance of clot formation at the stent site. Also, unless it's an emergency, patients should avoid other surgeries for a whole year after stent placement. Stopping clopidrogrel to accommodate an operation significantly raises the risk of stent-related complications developing.

Side effects associated with clopidogrel are similar to those caused by other antiplatelet agents: an increased tendency for bruising and an increased risk of bleeding.

Do Stents Have Any Side Effects?

There's no evidence that stents cause allergic reactions or that the immune system treats them as foreign objects. As best we can tell, stents are biologically inert. Stent placement essentially poses the same risks as angioplasty does: artery wall injury at the deployment site, renal insufficiency due to excessive use of contrast dye, stroke and heart attack due to dislodgement of atherosclerotic debris, soreness at the insertion point, and vessel damage.

The injury at the stent deployment site can manifest as coronary artery dissection (a tear in the artery) or coronary rupture (a hole in the artery causing blood leakage into the pericardial space). Both are uncommon occurrences. Other possible complications include coronary artery embolism, which occurs when a particle of plaque is dislodged and travels downstream into progressively more slender coronary arteries. Trapped in a narrower artery, the particle can cause a blood flow obstruction that results in heart attack. Abrupt vessel closure is a possibility, but that too is an uncommon event.

Are Angioplasty and Stenting a Complete Solution to Blood Vessel Narrowing?

Keep in mind two facts about angioplasty and stenting: first, they don't make you safe from heart attack; second, they improve quality of life, but they don't extend it. Thus far, the research has shown that stent implantation in a coronary artery does not reduce the incidence of heart attack; nor does it prolong life. The only proven role of angioplasty and stenting has been in reducing severity of chest discomfort associated with artery narrowing. But this can be important in terms of quality of life, particularly for patients who have persistent chest pain or in those who are too sick to undergo open-heart surgery.

Coronary Artery Bypass Graft Surgery

Thousands of coronary artery bypass graft (CABG) surgeries are performed yearly in the United States, making it one of the most frequently performed major operations. Bypass surgery involves opening up the rib cage by cutting through the breastbone (sternum) to expose the heart. This procedure is called sternotomy. The bypass procedure is made possible by use of a heart-lung machine (also called a cardiopulmonary bypass machine), a device that performs the functions of those organs during the surgery. To help protect the heart during bypass surgery, the heart is cooled by bathing it in a chilled, sterile solution.

To perform a bypass, blood vessel segments are taken ("harvested") from locations in the chest, arm, or leg, and relocated to a point just beyond the narrowed portion of a diseased coronary artery. The vessel segment that bypasses a coronary (heart) artery is called a graft; hence, the clinical name of the procedure: coronary artery bypass graft surgery.

Vessel segments used for bypass surgery vary in length from five to ten centimeters. To achieve a bypass, one end of a harvested vessel segment is most typically sewn into the aorta, the body's Alaskan pipeline, and the other onto the coronary artery, just slightly beyond ("downstream" from) its narrowed section.

From Which Parts of the Body Are Vessel Segments Harvested for Grafting?

Vessel segments may be taken from a number of places throughout the body.

Saphenous Grafts. Veins harvested for grafting are usually from a saphenous vein in the leg. Saphenous veins run vertically up the inside of the thighs, coursing near the groin. The cut ends of the donor vein are tied off, and blood gets rerouted through collateral vessels in the leg.

Patients who undergo a saphenous vein graft harvest may experience postoperative swelling in that leg as the blood makes an effort to reroute itself back to the heart. (The swelling is the result of the blood "pooling.") Other potential harvest effects include pain, infection at the harvest site, and altered sensation in the leg because of severed nerves. In general, mobility is not affected. Over time, the leg swelling decreases in most patients, but it's common to have some degree of lingering swelling and sensation loss. When swelling persists, patients are encouraged to wear compression stockings, which help minimize pooling by improving venous return, the process of routing blood back to the heart.

Did You Know?

Saphenous vein harvesting has advanced in its surgical technique. Endovascular harvesting, as the name suggests, utilizes an endoscope to harvest the vein segment. An endoscope is a small flexible tube with a light on the end, enabling the surgeon to visualize at a distance from the entry point to the skin. This permits smaller incisions as the endoscope is slipped under the skin to isolate and detach the vein. The recovery is sooner with less pain, risk of infection, and earlier mobility.

Mammary Arteries. In the chest, two excellent sources of vessel harvesting are the right and left internal mammary arteries (RIMA and LIMA). The LIMA is the most commonly used vessel for CABG, in part because of its strategic proximity to the heart. A LIMA bypass requires just one connection, rather than two, so there is no segment harvesting. It's close enough to the heart so that one end can be detached and then reattached to a narrowed artery on the front or side of the cardiac surface. The other option involves using a "free" mammary artery: a vessel segment removed from the LIMA or RIMA and connected to both the aorta and the coronary artery coursing on the heart's surface.

The right and left internal mammary arteries run vertically on each side of the heart, parallel with the sternum and just beneath the rib cage. Although we don't understand why, the LIMA and RIMA rarely develop significant atherosclerosis but provide reliable blood flow for decades. Once the LIMA and/or RIMA are rerouted, other arteries within the vicinity of the ribcage are able to assume their function.

How Long Can Grafted Vessels Last?

How long a graft effectively functions after surgery depends on the origin of the vessel segment, the skill of the cardiothoracic surgeon, and how much atherosclerotic disease has affected the area beyond the graft.

Remember, arteries send blood away from the heart; veins route the blood back to it. Since these vessels perform different functions, they're structurally different in key ways. Veins are designed to perform a low-pressure function, while arteries perform a higher-pressure function because they have to get the blood out to all tissues and propel its return through the veins. One way to think about this is to consider the difference between the work required to walk up a stairway or steep hill compared to the work required to make your way back down the incline. It takes significantly more effort to go up than it does to come down. For arteries, life is a constant uphill effort, but they're built to handle it.

Surgical success and graft longevity also depend in large part on the careful placement of the vessel segment. When a garden hose is twisted or kinked, water flow is significantly affected. The same thing happens with a bypass graft, so the segment has to be free of twists and kinks when it's grafted to the artery surface. This will ensure proper blood flow and graft function over time.

Of course, patient behavior after bypass surgery also is key to graft longevity. Obviously, grafts last longer in patients who manage their cholesterol levels, keep their blood pressure low, and quit smoking.

Saphenous Vein Grafts. Saphenous veins can be problematic when they serve as bypass grafts because they often suffer the same fate as diseased coronary arteries—they develop multiple areas of protruding plaques, some of which are prone to rupture or impede blood flow to the point of causing a heart attack. In some cases, using a saphenous vein for bypass is like replacing a clogged pipe with one that will eventually become more clogged.

Over time, when a saphenous vein is used as an arterial graft in CABG, the vein begins acting like an artery (arterialized) and becomes more muscular because its workload (and pressure inside it) has increased. Something about this process traumatizes the graft, making it more prone to atherosclerosis than internal mammary arteries in the ten years after surgery. Fifty percent of saphenous vein grafts at ten years will develop plaque buildup that causes significant narrowing. On the other hand, a very small percentage of saphenous vein grafts remain pristine after ten years.

Unfortunately, in some people with multiple blockages requiring four or five bypasses, utilizing saphenous vein grafts is a necessity. After all, only one or two IMA (internal mammary arteries) grafts are available.

Internal Mammary Artery Grafts. Grafts fashioned from an internal mammary artery have proved to be longer lasting and most effective. While we don't understand completely why the LIMA and RIMA grafts are devoid of significant atherosclerosis, the belief is that the physical structure of the grafts keeps them clear. The vessels are basically straight and have few large branch points, which means blood flow is smooth (laminar) and less likely to exert significant stress on the endothelial layer. Also, they're more muscular and able to accommodate the higher pressures of arterial blood flow without excess strain on the arterial wall.

How Does Grafting Affect Blood Flow?

In patients with diffuse coronary artery disease—where plaque has accumulated in many places in a coronary artery and caused many abnormally narrow passages—attaching a graft is the equivalent of having a brand-new four-lane highway suddenly converge into a one-lane dirt road with speed bumps. In the same way traffic would back up in that scenario, so too does blood streaming through a new bypass graft into the original artery.

The blood coursing through the graft (runoff) meets with significant resistance when it channels into the diseased and narrowed coronary artery. Blood flow is significantly impeded, resulting in blood stagnation in the graft. This increases the likelihood of clotting and graft failure due to the stalled blood flow. Premature graft closure can occur over hours to days.

Diffuse coronary artery disease is a problematic condition that can be difficult to treat. Unlike a tight blockage or narrowing in a single location, diffusely diseased coronary arteries demonstrate multiple blockages in succession. Some cardiologists liken diffuse disease to having a tiny string of pearls lining the artery. Each pearl represents protruding plaque that can impede blood flow. An artery with diffuse disease is very difficult to manage with stenting as no stent is long enough to address the totality of the blockages. Placing multiple stents end to end creates a scenario where there is a high likelihood of reblockage or possibly thrombosis and abrupt vessel closure. For those patients being considered for CABG, it's equally difficult for the cardiothoracic surgeon to place a graft because there's no good location for attaching it. The cardiothoracic surgeon wants to increase the blood supply through the diseased artery but also wants to minimize the likelihood of stagnation.

Clotting and graft closure due to diffuse disease and impaired downstream blood flow can occur in both an internal mammary artery and a saphenous vein graft.

Can Bypass Surgery Prolong Life?

To reiterate: CABG success depends upon surgical skill in terms of the graft site attachment, how well blood flows beyond the graft site (dictated by the size of the artery), and the extent of "downstream" coronary artery disease. But unlike angioplasty and stenting, successful coronary artery bypass graft surgery has been demonstrated to prolong life in certain groups of bypass patients. These include patients with:

- Severe "three-vessel" coronary artery disease (three coronary arteries with advanced obstructive plaque)
- Left main coronary artery disease
- Severe three-vessel coronary artery disease and reduced heart function

What Is Recovery from Bypass Surgery Like?

Most patients who have undergone bypass surgery will be prescribed aspirin; some will go on warfarin, particularly patients who have had atrial arrhythmias before the bypass or were complicated by it. Both medications are used to minimize the risk of blood clotting: aspirin within the heart arteries and bypass grafts and warfarin within the heart itself.

• • • *Fast Fact* • • •

Remember that warfarin has not been proven to be beneficial for preventing coronary atherosclerosis or reducing heart attack and cardiac death rates in patients with coronary artery disease, including those patients who have undergone CABG.

• • •

Compared with recovery from angioplasty and stenting, bypass surgery recuperation can last several months. Immediately after the procedure, most patients stay in the hospital a minimum of five days.

In general, a patient can regain about 80 percent of preoperative strength within one to two months after surgery, provided the prescribed postsurgical diet and exercise regimens are carefully followed. Also, though it may seem obvious, smoking should be avoided because in addition to damaging the lungs, it damages arteries, promotes atherosclerosis, and hinders the body's ability to heal.

Part of the recovery prescription—perhaps the most important part—involves enrolling in a supervised cardiac rehabilitation program. Such programs possess the inherent expertise necessary to create individualized exercise regimens and goals. The point of cardiac rehabilitation is not to prepare you for the Olympics, but to safely get you moving after surgery, accelerate the healing process, and give you a healthy lifestyle to be maintained for the remainder of your life. This includes eating a heart-healthy diet and engaging in regular exercise. In an effective cardiac rehabilitation program, you'll work closely with clinicians to design a plan that works best for you and your lifestyle.

Over time, CABG patients may undergo a corrective or "repeat" procedure to manage progressive coronary atherosclerosis. This could mean another bypass surgery or angioplasty and stenting of a narrowed coronary artery, including a graft artery.

What Keeps the Body Alive While You Operate on the Heart?

Traditional bypass surgery uses a heart-lung machine, an indispensable tool that takes on the tasks normally performed by the heart and lungs: pumping blood, removing carbon dioxide and other waste products from the blood, and then reoxygenating it. Deoxygenated (and carbon-dioxide-rich) blood is siphoned from the right atrium and redirected to the heart-lung machine; as it leaves the machine, the cleaned and oxygenated blood is channeled into the ascending aorta and from there circulates throughout the body.

The system also warms or cools blood to help control body temperature. The machine permits a surgeon to work on a still and essentially bloodless heart, rather than a beating one. This helps optimize surgical results and minimize the risk of inadvertent injury.

Without the heart-lung machine, open-heart surgery options would be quite limited. But the complex apparatus also accounts for some of the risk associated with bypass surgery. To get the machine up and running, the ascending aorta and right atrium must be punctured so the machine's tubes (cannulas) can be attached to the aorta and atrium. The processing that blood undergoes in a heart-lung machine can create blood clots that cause heart attack, stroke, or kidney failure, so patients must be given anticlotting medicines. So despite the countless lives it has saved, the heart-lung machine is not devoid of risk.

Can Surgeons Operate on a Beating Heart?

A procedure called beating heart surgery eliminates the need for the heart-lung machine and its cannulas. Under this bypass procedure, the heart continues beating, and blood flow remains normally routed. With the help of special tools, heart surgeons stabilize and immobilize sections of the heart to minimize tissue movement caused by heart pumping and contraction. Beta blockers are also administered to slow heart rate and reduce the vigor of heart contractions. Beating heart surgery can significantly lower the risk of clotting, and patients who undergo the procedure may also recuperate faster than those who undergo traditional bypass.

Not surprisingly, beating heart surgery demands significant training and great skill, both because of the surgical tools used and the challenge of attaching grafts to tissue that is in motion. So it's still used selectively. The ideal candidates for this operation are patients whose blocked arteries are on the front of the heart, which is more accessible to surgeons.

Are There Less Invasive Methods of Heart Surgery?

There are heart surgery strategies utilizing less invasive procedures that eliminate the need for opening the rib cage at the sternum. With these approaches, small incisions are made on the side of the chest and between the ribs to gain access to the heart. The goal is to minimize trauma to the body (thoracic cage or chest cavity) so that recuperation is faster and less onerous for the patient. Compared with traditional heart surgery, less invasive surgery results in less bleeding, a lower risk of infection, shorter hospitals stays, less severe scarring, and a quicker return to normal activities. Less invasive surgery utilizing a surgeon-guided robot is also currently selectively deployed. This may also prove to ease recovery, avoiding the need of opening the midchest through the sternum.

Did You Know?

The term *minimally invasive surgery* suggests that open heart surgery may be categorized other than as a major operation. I prefer the term *less invasive heart surgery*. Particularly when the patient is deeply anesthetized and the heart is stopped, that qualifies as a major operation with inherent risk, independent of the mode of chest cavity access.

What's Best for You

Patients who have access to heart centers using these new bypass surgery techniques should discuss with their physician the procedure that best fits their needs. Here are a few fundamental criteria that should guide your questioning:

1. Opt for the best operation possible: one that's safe and effective, allows the surgeon optimal exposure to the heart surface, and is most likely to achieve a lasting outcome.

2. Don't sacrifice the quality of the operation with the sole goal of shortening your recovery and possibly setting yourself up for a repeat operation in a shorter period. Beating heart surgery or robotic surgery should be chosen only if the surgeon has the experience and proven track record with these procedures.

3. Should you decide in favor of a less invasive or robotic approach, ask the surgeon who will perform the procedure whether he or she has significant experience with it, and verify that the procedure produces a satisfactory rate of positive outcomes. In other words, the procedure should have a great record of success at the center using it.

Do not underestimate the emotional challenges of open heart surgery. When faced with a major operation, denial and depression both enter the picture. In fact, a fair number of patients develop a lingering depression after open heart surgery, many adopting a "why me" viewpoint. It is important to know that bypass surgery represents a new beginning, a new opportunity for the rest of your life. I often refer to it with my patients as a "speed bump" with a greater than 95 percent success rate. Is there time and discomfort involved? Absolutely! Do the benefits outweigh the risks? Absolutely! This is where an open and trusting doctor-patient relationship will pay huge dividends. The emotional aspects generally sort themselves out over time as the recovery proceeds in a positive direction coupled with the patient enrolling in a cardiac rehabilitation program. Tangible improvements in activity level and less reliance on pain medication collectively support both the physical and emotional recovery of CABG patients.

Ray's Story

Ray was lying on his back on a gurney, minutes away from being wheeled into a cardiothoracic operating room for surgery that would cut open his chest and either save him or kill him. The night before, a priest had administered last rites. Ray was not so scared for himself as for his wife, three sons, two daughters-in-law, and two new grandchildren. He'd lived a good life—they all had. Nothing fancy or extravagant, but hard work had paid off for all of them, and until now, they'd been blessed with good health. Ray had done his best during the weeks leading up to this moment to preoccupy everyone, to keep things light, to keep doing what they did as a family—engaging one another, debating, ribbing. It was just a diversion. Ray refused to let things get maudlin. But minutes before surgery, reality and mortality were tough to avoid.

Four weeks earlier, on August 15, 1995, Ray had arrived at a heart center in Cleveland, by helicopter, from Elkins

Hospital, a small medical center in tiny Elkins, West Virginia. Ray's family lived in Cleveland, but they owned a small A-frame at Black Bear Resort, adjacent to the Canaan Valley Ski Resort. Every summer, the A-frame was the gathering place for family reunions. It was a time to reconnect with loved ones, take in the scenery, relax with people they cherished.

In the back of the A-frame was a deck and, to one side, a hot tub. It was a little while before dinner and things were comparatively quiet, so Ray decided to catch up on his academic duties (in addition to running his own consulting firm, he was a professor of management in an MBA program) while enjoying a soak.

Ray made himself a highball, grabbed a stack of exams, glided happily out onto the deck, slid into the hot tub, and began working his way through the papers. The combination of the setting, the medicinal warmth of the water, the ritual of doing a job he loved, and the sensation caused by the chilled, quenching drink put Ray into a wonderful, relaxed state. He was pretty much in heaven. After a while, he noticed some tingling and numbness in his left arm. But that was nothing new, really, inasmuch as he'd almost lost part of the arm (and part of his face) years earlier in a freak accident with a sliding glass door. Ever since, the arm had sporadically acted up. In fact, soaking in the hot tub seemed to work wonders for it. He shook his arm vigorously and tried to focus on the grading.

Then something really odd happened. He was staring at a student's exam when suddenly he had the sensation that his brain function had somehow become frozen. For . . . some . . . inexplicable . . . reason . . . he . . . couldn't . . . think . . . fast.

This set off alarms that something obviously was not right. Minutes before, he would have simply stood up and climbed out of the tub. But now he was engaged in a labored, sluggish debate about whether . . . to . . . extricate . . . himself . . . from . . . the . . . tub . . . or . . . stay . . . put.

It seemed like forever before he reached a decision—get out of the tub! Fine, he was out. But now he began debating whether to towel off. What in God's name was going on here? Then he figured it out. I'm having a stroke. Fine, Dr. Ray; now, just tell Betty. *He yelled to his wife.* "Betty, call 911! I'm having a stroke!" *She yelled back,* "And what if they say you've just been in the hot tub too long? I warned you about this." *Even so, she came out to the deck and found her husband standing there, a towel hanging uselessly from his hand, sweating profusely, but looking very much alive.* "Betty, call 911. I'm having a stroke," *he repeated. She called.*

Having convinced himself that he was having a stroke, Ray tried to convince everybody else of this, beginning with his family members, who rushed to his side and ministered to him while they waited for the medics to arrive. Then he tried to convert the paramedics, who determined within seconds that it was actually his heart and proceeded to inject him with clot-degrading drugs. "I'm fine," *Ray insisted throughout the one-hour ambulance ride over three small mountain ranges.*

At Elkins Hospital, he tried selling the stroke diagnosis to the emergency-room docs as they went through their clinical paces. They weren't buying. Nor was the cardiologist, who by Ray's estimate, looked to be just shy of 20 years old. Ray was the only one who thought it was a stroke. How could they all be so ignorant? *Ray wondered.* If I was having a heart attack, I'd feel like I was having a heart attack. I'd have chest pain. I wouldn't be able to breathe. I'd be knocking on death's door. So what if I can't stop sweating? I was in a hot tub, for God's sake. I feel fine!

After he got more test results, the Elkins cardiologist told Ray they'd be transferring him to another hospital in the area, one that was better equipped to deal with such serious cardiac cases. The plan was to transfer him ASAP, whether Ray believed the diagnosis or not (later, the "big-city" cardiologist who took over Ray's care would tell him that the Elkins staff "did everything we would have done to manage the situation"). Ray felt nervous about getting care from a hospital so far from home. The cardiologist explained that he'd never make it through an eight-hour ambulance ride, and the hospital wasn't authorized to life-flight him in. Ray thought about this a few seconds. He may have disagreed with the diagnosis, but he certainly didn't want to die. And if he really was on the edge, he wanted to be at a hospital in his own city. So he handed over his American Express card and said, "Get me on the helicopter."

But even at the heart center in Cleveland, Ray was still in denial about his condition. His heart had suffered the equivalent of a blow from a hammer. Four arteries were severely clogged, he had extensive scar tissue from the heart attack, and he was showing signs of heart failure. The whole organ was extremely fragile. Ray was fragile. Angioplasty and stenting wouldn't be enough to put him back on track. He would be on numerous medications, and his quality of life would take a nosedive because he'd have to avoid all strenuous and energetic activity. His status also put him at high risk for complications from open-heart surgery. On the other hand, surgery just might save his life.

The more Ray thought about it, the more he believed that he had no choice but to choose surgery, because doing nothing could just as easily kill him.

Two members of the cardiothoracic surgical team wheeled Ray into the operating room. Unbeknownst to him, in addition to bringing changes of clothes with them, his three sons had also brought dark suits. His wife had been advised privately that Ray would be lucky to survive the surgery, so she put the word out to her sons. Ray, who by this time had accepted the seriousness of his situation, set down on paper detailed instructions for his memorial service, offering guidance on who should speak and what music should be played. Should things not go well, the plan was to keep him alive long enough to allow everyone to say their goodbyes.

Aftermath

Eleven years after he looked into the eyes of family members for what could have been the last time, Ray is alive and well. During the bypass, surgeons made an incision from Ray's neck to his belly button to provide access to his heart, as well as incisions in both legs that ran from his groin to his ankles, so that the grafts that would save his life could be harvested. He woke up from the surgery and remembered not to panic when he couldn't open his eyes because they were taped shut. He couldn't talk because he had a garden hose coursing through his gullet. He spent weeks sleeping in a wing-backed chair because lying down made breathing impossible. He began his slow but determined crawl back to life with the help of the heart center's cardiac rehabilitation program, in which he continues to participate. He's back at work and he tries to make every minute count.

Ray never smoked and remains an avid exerciser. He dodged a bullet, but he knows that things could change at any time. Ray's mother, for instance, a smoker, dropped dead from a heart attack at age 62. Two weeks after Ray's brother-in-law retired from nearly two decades of directing a prestigious medical association, the 62-year-old was dead from a heart attack. He'd been out riding his bike, relishing the beautiful weather and looking forward to the next phase of what he assumed would be a satisfying, fulfilling experience of growing old. Ray's brother-in-law never knew he had heart disease. "You have experiences like that," says Ray, who was also 62 when he had his heart attack, "and it's hard not to wonder, *How did that happen to him, and I'm still here?*"

No matter how old you are, there's always something you want to live for—the next party, the next grandchild, the next graduation. Eventually, you must face the fact that you're not going to be able to show up for every new occasion. But until then, like Ray, you can keep showing up, keep celebrating life. And coronary artery bypass graft surgery can help make that possible.

Chapter 9

Exercise

E xercising on a regular basis has several benefits for improving heart health. Over time, regular exercise can:

- Help raise levels of good cholesterol
- Lower blood pressure
- Increase energy levels
- Increase muscle mass
- Help maintain bone density
- Improve emotional health

Exercise alone isn't a perfect weight management or weight loss tool, but when combined with healthy changes in diet, weight loss and weight management are much more likely. For sure, most people struggle to make lifestyle changes part of their daily routines. But in addition to the aforementioned health benefits, exercise can help you reduce or eliminate the need for medications commonly used to help manage heart disease. These include blood pressure medications and cholesterol-lowering agents.

How Much Exercise Will Make the Difference?

Initiating, and then sticking to a regular exercise program, is the most important immediate change you can make to positively

Did You Know?

Exercising at a moderate pace grants a higher likelihood of you sustaining your exercise regime. If it is a punitive experience, dreading your next workout may work in the short term but not in the long term.

affect your emotional and physical health. But an Olympic effort isn't required. Very beneficial results can come from thirty minutes of quality exercise (jogging, running, swimming, jumping rope, aerobics, yoga, Pilates, tennis, ice skating, rollerblading, cycling, skiing, rock climbing, and even brisk walking) performed four to five days a week.

Although the ideal goal would be to exercise seven days a week, the most important principle to understand is that some exercise is better than no exercise. Any exercise that gets you moving—on a consistent basis—and safely raises the heart rate for a sustained period is beneficial. For men and women, weight-bearing exercises (walking, running, weight lifting, hiking, rock climbing, jumping rope, aerobics) are also beneficial because they help maintain bone and muscle mass.

Regardless of the exercise, one key to success is to begin slowly, so that the first few efforts are positive and rewarding rather than punitive and distressing. Forget the old saw "No pain, no gain." A positive experience at the outset, particularly for individuals who have been sedentary for some time, increases the likelihood that you'll return to the exercise program and continue it for a long time. Ease into a program, but stay focused and disciplined. Give yourself a pat on the back, and look forward to making exercise part of lasting lifestyle change.

As to exertion levels, while you exercise, you should be able to carry on a reasonable conversation without gasping for air. For example, if you're running on a treadmill, riding a stationary bike, or cycling outdoors, and someone asks you a question, you should be able to answer it. If you're too winded to answer or unable to complete a sentence, you're overdoing it and you need to back off a bit. In general, this is true for everyone, irrespective of size.

Where Do I Begin?

If you've been sedentary for some time and are not in the greatest physical condition, it's important to:

- See a physician to make sure there are no "silent" health concerns that warrant treatment or further investigation, such as high blood pressure, high cholesterol, or an abnormal resting electrocardiogram
- Work with a physician to develop a "beginning" exercise prescription

Despite their enthusiasm or good intentions, many patients don't have the knowledge to create their own safe and effective exercise program. The best way to achieve this is to work with

Consider This

I am frequently asked by my patients what is the best level or degree of exercise. I think exercising aerobically for thirty minutes continuously five days per week is best. The intensity of the exercise should be gauged by your breathing. At maximal exercise, you should be able to speak in reasonably full sentences. If your speech is fragmented or significantly labored, then you should back off a bit and resume your exercise at a more intense level when you are better conditioned.

an experienced preventive cardiology program, so ask your physician about hooking up with one. These programs typically have an experienced exercise physiologist on staff and can develop a customized exercise program for you.

What Does My Heart Rate Have to Do with Exercise?

Sustained elevation of your heart rate during exercise, adjusted for age, as illustrated by the heart rate calculation chart (see box below), is the key to cardiovascular risk reduction. This is far more important than whether exercise is transforming you physically. Aerobic conditioning that is derived from a sustained exercise

Calculating Your Target Heart Rate

This heart rate calculation tool illustrates how adult men and women can determine age-adjusted heart rates (heart beats per minute) that are suitable for safe, effective exercise sessions.

For women:

226 minus your age = age-adjusted maximum heart rate; multiply by 75 percent.

Example: 55-year-old woman

$226 - 55 = 171 \times .75 = 128.25$

Target heart rate goal during exercise: 128 beats per minute

For men:

220 minus your age = age-adjusted maximum heart rate; multiply by 75 percent

Example: 55-year-old man

$220 - 55 = 165 \times .75 = 123.75$

Target heart rate goal during exercise: 124 beats per minute program will lower your resting heart rate and blood pressure. These two achievements alone will give you more energy, improve your sense of well-being, and build self-esteem. But most important, they'll help reduce the risk of future cardiovascular events like heart attack or stroke.

Patients without diagnosed coronary artery disease should try to exercise for thirty minutes and at a level that elevates normal heart rate (pulse rate) and breathing (respiratory rate). The American Heart Association recommends that during any moderate to vigorous aerobic activity, you maintain 50 to 75 percent of your maximum heart rate.

Is It Safe to Exercise If I Am at Risk for a Heart Attack?

Those who want to start exercising but possess a host of risk factors (heart disease history, high blood pressure, overweight, smoking) or have been sedentary for many years are urged to see a physician before they begin, even if they feel fine. The absence of heart disease symptoms doesn't mean the absence of heart disease.

Age should also guide your decision to see a physician. In men, the prevalence of coronary artery disease really picks up starting at age 45; in women, prevalence picks up significantly during the postmenopausal years. In fact, this is the time when women really catch up to men in terms of coronary artery disease incidence and heart attacks. And they catch up rapidly.

People who are sedentary, at risk for coronary artery disease, and in the aforementioned age groups need to establish an exercise capacity before they start because sedentary people who suddenly start exercising often have goals that are beyond their capabilities. In other words, they start out too hard and too fast. This increases their risk for exercise-induced myocardial ischemia (insufficient oxygen delivery during strenuous activity) or even an exercise-related abnormal heart rhythm.

Therefore, seeing a primary care physician or cardiologist before taking up exercise, at least for a screening exam, is wise. At that time, a decision can be made about whether stress testing is warranted. This test screens for asymptomatic (symptomless) coronary artery disease and heart dysfunction such as previously undiagnosed heart muscle weakening and the possibility of a prior silent heart attack. A stress test also identifies exercise capacity, and that information can serve as the basis for creating a safe and effective exercise program.

Exercise Tips.

1. Exercise within your own comfortable limits.
2. Start slow; progress gradually.
3. Make exercise a lifestyle change, not a passing interest.
4. Incorporate exercise into your daily schedule, and honor it.

Chapter 10

Preventive Cardiology and Rehabilitation

Effective cardiovascular health management means preventing heart disease. A preventive cardiology and rehabilitation program is designed to address this challenge by helping you make lifestyle changes that will improve overall health and, in particular, heart health.

Whether you are at high risk for cardiovascular disease or heart attack, or are recovering from a cardiac event or intervention such as stenting or bypass surgery, a preventive cardiology program will help improve physical strength and mobility, build energy levels, lower blood pressure, decrease cholesterol levels, improve diabetes control, spur weight loss, and beat nicotine dependence.

Your Cardiology Program

Any cardiology program—whether designed for the postoperative patient or the high-risk patient—has three overarching objectives:

- Improving overall heart and cardiovascular health
- Preventing the occurrence and/or progression of cardio-vascular disease
- Reducing the risk of a heart attack, stroke, or need for future cardiovascular intervention

However, the way in which you meet these objectives is determined by your approach.

Who Will Design My Cardiology Program?

An effective preventive cardiology and rehabilitation program uses experts from an array of disciplines: cardiovascular medicine, endocrinology, hypertension, internal medicine, exercise physiology, psychology, and nutrition therapy. These experts collaborate on developing individualized strategies for diet, exercise, and lifestyle change. A comprehensive preventive cardiology and rehabilitation program also offers guidance about smoking cessation, diet, exercise, blood pressure, weight, cholesterol levels, and stress management.

• • • Fast Fact • • •

I have found that a healthcare team comprised of experts from differing areas of expertise adds significantly to health outcomes. That's because no one patient is the same. We all are unique and therefore possess our own set of health challenges be it, for example, cardiovascular, diabetic, or orthopedic. All of these may impact the design and implementation of a cardiac rehabilitation program, best achieved through a multidisciplinary approach.

• • •

Once a plan is created, the patient works closely with preventive cardiology staff, who help manage the regimen, offer encouragement and feedback, monitor health status, and document progress and goal achievement. All sessions, in fact, should be medically supervised by registered nurses or certified rehabilitation specialists such as exercise physiologists. Patients typically collaborate on these individualized plans with physicians and registered dietitians.

What Will My Cardiology Program Include?

The key components of a preventive cardiology and rehabilitation program should include risk factor evaluation; cardiovascular disease education (including heart anatomy and the emotional challenges associated with heart disease); diet and exercise plans; one-on-one guidance from certified preventive cardiology staff; access to specialists such as endocrinologists, licensed dietitians, and psychotherapists; and regular monitoring of benchmarks such as weight, blood pressure, cholesterol levels, exercise duration, and reinvolvement in day-to-day routines.

Cardiac rehabilitation usually begins in the hospital and continues throughout recovery. There are typically three phases.

Phase I. Phase I begins during hospitalization, where you're educated about the recovery process and learn how to manage risk factors and reduce the likelihood of future cardiac events. Exercise also begins during hospitalization.

Phase II. Phase II begins immediately after hospitalization and involves on-site visits by the patient to the outpatient preventive cardiology facility. It also involves additional education about lifestyle changes, introduction to heart-healthy diet and exercise regimens, training on exercise techniques, and monitoring of progress.

Phase III. Phase III is the lifelong "maintenance" portion of the program. During this phase, you use what you've learned to proactively manage heart disease. This can be performed on your own or this can be part of either an individual or group exercise program.

• • • *Fast Fact* • • •

Many of my patients find an ongoing structured exercise program beneficial in terms of maintaining a long-term exercise commitment. Relationships are formed with other participants, and the exercise routine proves energizing both physically and emotionally.

• • •

What Makes a Cardiology Program Successful?

Success of a cardiovascular prevention and rehabilitation plan depends on several factors. The plan has to be carefully tailored to fit a patient's health status, risk factors, living situation, and goals and objectives. Ideally, the patient's physician is involved in the plan and helps monitor progress on a regular basis, paying particular attention to cholesterol levels and management of chronic diseases such as diabetes and high blood pressure. The plan has to be financially feasible and realistic—goals have to be attainable in a reasonable period, and exercise regimens should fit a patient's physical status and schedule.

Success also depends on a patient's willingness to work with the preventive cardiology program. For some patients, making lifestyle changes isn't easy; they find themselves moving in fits and starts. They may have trouble adjusting to a regular exercise program and improved diet, or have schedules that make regular exercise a difficult proposition. Nicotine's pull may be too tempting. So it's up to everyone involved to be creative about helping the patient persist in achieving goals, making lifestyle changes, and optimizing health.

Who Would Benefit from a Preventive Cardiology Program?

The range of patients who can benefit from a preventive cardiology and rehabilitation program is broad and includes those recovering from surgical and interventional procedures such as:

- Angioplasty and stenting
- Coronary artery bypass grafting
- Valve repair or replacement
- Aortic aneurysm repair or replacement
- Heart transplant
- Implantation of pacemakers or internal defibrillators (ICDs)

A good preventive cardiology program should also focus upon a range of cardiac conditions such as congestive heart failure, arrhythmia (abnormal heart rhythm), hemodynamic (blood pressure) disorders, and other cardiovascular-related problems. Most health insurance plans offer some level of coverage for preventive cardiology and rehabilitation programs—check your plan to find out what is covered. Check with your physician to see if what you are pursuing is safe.

Remember Ray from chapter 9? I first met Ray in 1994 at the time of his acute hospitalization after his heart attack and episode of congestive heart failure. His condition was tenuous, having suffered a large heart attack, and there was uncertainty if he was going to survive. If he survived we were not certain for how long. One thing that was clear to me right from the start was that Ray had an immensely supportive family. I also remember being impressed with Ray's will to live. He faced heart surgery but viewed it as a necessary step to resume the rest of his life.

As you recall, Ray recovered spectacularly from his open-heart surgery, and with the exception of the placement of an implantable cardiac defibrillator, Ray has not been rehospitalized for the past 14 years. His cholesterol levels are outstanding, his weight is lower, and his diabetes is under much better control on a reduced medication regime.

So, what has been Ray's secret to this success? I would identify his attitude and supportive family as first and foremost. Provided the closeness and genuine love of his family, Ray has a true will to live. His attitude is outstanding, and he has garnered the confidence over time that he has regained his health, and he anticipates that he will continue to do well. A close second is his commitment to exercise. This has been unwavering since enrolling in his local cardiac rehabilitation program shortly after his bypass surgery. He successfully completed Phase II cardiac rehabilitation six weeks after his open heart surgery and has remained in Phase III for nearly 15 years. He has incorporated exercise as part of his daily routine, encourages others to do so, and is a true success story when it comes to a positive attitude and a disciplined approach to healthy living through regular aerobic exercise.

Chapter 11

Choosing a Physician

One of the best things you can do regarding choosing a physician to care for your heart health is to be proactive. Don't wait until something bad happens to start looking for the right doctor. Take stock of your health, family history, and risk factors, and be honest with yourself. If all the indicators point to any degree of heart disease risk, then take some time to determine who is the most qualified—and available—to care for you should the need arise.

Start by asking your primary care physician for a recommended cardiologist. And ask family members and trusted friends or acquaintances, particularly those who have heart disease or are at high risk for it.

Plenty of patients assess a physician's ability based on personality and rapport. While these are important attributes and can make for positive, mutually rewarding clinical interactions, your focus should be on experience and outcomes. A pleasant, affable personality is a bonus but certainly not a requirement for outstanding medical care.

What Should I Look for in a Physician?

Choosing a physician, including a cardiologist, is an extremely important decision. Of the many considerations, the most important are clinical experience (extent of training in a given specialty, where the training occurred, number of years practicing in that specialty, level of credentialing) and patient outcomes (how well patients fare under that physician's care in the wake of treatment or intervention). Board certification is an additional important factor. Don't be afraid to ask a doctor to provide verification of licensure, training, and board certification. If the doctor is insulted by such inquiries or does not respond to them, consider finding another doctor.

The due diligence involved in assessing qualifications and expertise, however, shouldn't begin and end with the physician you ultimately choose for your care because, over time, you may need guidance and care from different types of cardiologists as well as nonheart specialists. This makes it important to size up the level of expertise and experience among those with whom you and your physician will be collaborating. The most effective medical care for chronic disease involves collaboration among physicians from different specialties. You'll want to make sure the physician you choose is part of, or has direct access to, a multi-disciplinary team.

For instance, suppose you experience chest pain or discomfort and decide to seek out a cardiologist. The cardiologist you choose may be a noninvasive cardiologist (one who does not perform invasive procedures such as angioplasty and stenting), one whose expertise involves diagnosing heart disease and managing it with medicine. If your heart disease at some point warrants intervention, you want to be confident that your cardiologist can refer you quickly to a trusted, experienced colleague who is skilled in interventional cardiology, electrophysiology, or cardiothoracic surgery. If, in addition to your heart disease, you have diabetes or high blood pressure, you'll want access to skilled internists and endocrinologists. In short, you need access to a highly skilled team of physicians representing a broad range of clinical expertise.

One way to identify an adequate or high level of multidisciplinary care is to first start with a hospital or medical center known for its expertise in managing heart disease. One handy source for identifying these is the U.S. News/American Hospital Association Directory, which rates expertise in an array of clinical specialties. The list is updated every year and available online (*http://health. usnews.com/directories/hospital-directory/*).

Overall, you want to get information about credentials, experience, range of services offered, whether a center engages in research and education, level of patient satisfaction, and outcomes.

What Is "Outcomes Data," and Is It Important?

Outcomes data, also known as quality measures, are extremely important pieces of information relating to medical care and intervention. They provide information about complications associated with certain treatments or procedures as well as information on how successful they are in managing a condition and prolonging life. Useful outcomes data tell you about infection rates, side effects, length of hospital stay, the need for corrective or emergency care in the aftermath of a treatment or procedure, and death (mortality) rates.

If the medical center or hospital you are dealing with cannot or will not provide this information, move on to another one. It's also very important that information is presented for individual treatments and procedures. It doesn't matter how many heart attack patients a hospital has treated; what matters is the clinical experience of patients managed with medical therapy, angioplasty and stenting, bypass surgery, or some combination of these. What was the infection rate for patients undergoing bypass surgery? What percentage needed second operations? How long, on average, were patients hospitalized after surgery? What percentage of patients

Outcomes Data Online

An increasing number of medical centers are making outcomes data available in promotional materials and via the Internet. The Cleveland Clinic website features a special section devoted to educating patients about understanding and using outcomes data as well as presenting data about its own clinical experiences in cardiovascular medicine. The address for the site is *www.clevelandclinic.org*/quality. Two other valuable sources of guidance on these matters are MedlinePlus, a service of the U.S. National Library of Medicine and the National Institutes of Health, and the Agency for Healthcare Research and Quality, the lead federal agency charged with improving the quality, safety, efficiency, and effectiveness of health care for all Americans.

were living five years after surgery? Answers to these questions can help you determine which center is most likely to offer you the highest level of care.

The optimal patient-physician relationships are those in which you are comfortable in your physician's presence, you can confide in your doctor without reservation, and you are confident that he or she has the experience, skill, and dedication to provide, or seek out for you, the best care possible. Responsivity of your physician is another vitally important metric to assess. In addition to my office contact information, printing my email address on my business card and stationery has proved beneficial. I have found this to be an exceedingly efficient and timely mode of communication. Certainly, if one of my patients would like to speak to me, they have the option of calling my office or directly emailing me to request a return phone call.

Conclusion

The progress of contemporary cardiovascular medicine has been amazing. Who would have thought that we as cardiologists have at our disposal small wires with ultrasound transducers to directly image and characterize atherosclerotic plaque? Plus the ability to perform angioplasty and stent coronary artery blockages, reducing the need for open heart surgery. And let's not forget the refinements of open heart surgery including, most importantly, the reduced complication and death rates. More complex operations are occurring via smaller incisions and resulting in reduced recovery times.

Equally important is the advance in available medical therapy. First and foremost is the development and widespread use of statin medication to lower cholesterol and to stabilize plaque. Clopidogrel, administered after stent placement, has been shown to unequivocally reduce stent complications including thrombus formation.

These advancements are remarkable, but it's not time for complacency. The mechanical heart is still more theoretical than widely applied. Those patients with large heart attacks with significantly impaired heart function face an uncertain future. Cardiac transplantation is an outstanding alternative for some, but is severely limited by suitable organ availability.

On the horizon, the most promising new treatment option for heart attack patients is stem cell therapy. Advances are being made by directly injecting adult stem cells into damaged heart muscle with improved cardiac muscle perfusion and a modest improvement in heart function. This is an area of intense research both in the basic laboratory and also at the patient's bedside. When clinically available, stem cell therapy stands to make the largest clinical impact to date by regenerating damaged and scarred cardiac muscle.

Lastly, it is my hope that this book communicated the importance of your active role as a patient in your overall health. Many of you reading this book have either suffered a heart attack, almost certainly know someone who suffered a heart attack, or are trying to educate yourself to preempt your own heart attack. I believe the future of healthcare is disease preemption. Remain an active participant in your health. You stand to benefit greatly.

Appendix 1

Online Resources

Cleveland Clinic Heart and Vascular Institute:
www.clevelandclinic.org/heartcenter

Cleveland Clinic Quality and Safety Patient Institute:
www.clevelandclinic.org/quality

———

Agency for Healthcare Research and Quality:
www.ahrq.gov/consumer/guidetoq/index.html

American Heart Association:
www.americanheart.org

The Heart Truth:
www.nhlbi.nih.gov/health/hearttruth/index.htm

MedlinePlus:
www.nlm.nih.gov/medlineplus/choosingadoctororhealthcareservice.html

National Heart, Lung, and Blood Institute:
www.nhlbi.nih.gov

The National Coalition for Women with Heart Disease:
www.womenheart.org

U.S. News and World Report Hospital Directory Search:
www.usnews.com/usnews/health/hospitals/hosp_home.htm

WebMD:
www.webmd.com/

WebMD's "theheart.org":
www.theheart.org

Your Total Health—Heart Health:
http://yourtotalhealth.ivillage.com/heart-health

Appendix 2

Choosing a Heart-Healthy Diet

The foods below are recommended for people with congestive heart failure because these foods are typically low in salt, saturated fat, and cholesterol.* Learn to read food labels to help you choose more heart-healthy foods when you shop.

Fruits

- Fresh, canned, or frozen

Vegetables

- (Avoid sauce or flavor pouches, which add salt and fat. Canned is OK if unsalted or rinsed.)
- Fresh or frozen

Meats, Poultry, Fish

- Fresh or frozen fish (not breaded)
- Canned tuna and salmon (unsalted or rinsed)
- Chicken or turkey, both with the skin removed
- Lean cuts of beef, veal, pork, or lamb (trim away all fat)

---

* Heart-healthy foods are reproduced with permission of the American Heart Association, *www.americanheart.org* ©2006, American Heart Association.

Meat Substitutes
- Dried beans, peas, lentils (not canned)
- Tofu (soybean curd)

Nuts or Seeds
- (Eat nuts in small amounts because they're high in fat and calories.)
- Unsalted and dry-roasted, such as sunflower seeds, peanuts, almonds, and walnuts
- Unsalted peanut butter

Drinks: Fruit Juices; Fresh, Frozen, or Canned Drinks
- Canned low-sodium or no-salt-added tomato and vegetable juice
- Breakfast drink, powder or liquid (limit to 1 cup/day)
- Lemonade (frozen concentrate or fresh)

Other Drinks
- Tea and coffee in moderation
- Soy protein powder, soy milk

Dairy Choices
- (Choose 2–3 servings of these low-fat dairy products per day.)
- Liquid or dry milk (1 percent, ½ percent, fat-free or nonfat)
- Cottage cheese, dry curd (low sodium)
- Low-fat or part-skim cheeses, such as ricotta and mozzarella
- Neufchatel

Fats, Oils (Use any of these in small amounts.)

- Unsaturated vegetable oils like canola, olive, corn, cotton seed, peanut, safflower, soybean, and sunflower
- Low-sodium, low-fat salad dressing and mayonnaise
- Unsalted margarine with liquid vegetable oil as first ingredient

Breads, Cereals, Grains, Starches

- Pasta
- Rice (enriched white or brown)
- Starchy vegetables, such as corn, potatoes, green peas, etc. (not canned unless salt-free)
- Loaf bread and yeast rolls
- Homemade breads (with regular flour, not self-rising)
- Melba toast
- Matzo crackers
- Pita bread
- Taco shell, corn tortilla
- Cooked cereals, such as corn grits, farina (regular), oatmeal, oat bran, cream of rice, cream of wheat (avoid instant cereals)
- Puffed rice or wheat, shredded wheat, or any cereal with 100–150 mg of sodium (limit to 1 cup/day)
- Wheat germ (in small amounts)
- Unsalted, no-fat popcorn

Cooking Ingredients and Seasonings

- Corn starch, tapioca
- Cornmeal (not self-rising because of high salt content)
- Fresh or dried herbs, salt-free herb seasonings
- Regular white or whole-wheat flour (not self-rising)

- Fresh fruits and vegetables, such as lemons, limes, onions, celery, etc.
- Fresh garlic or ginger
- Louisiana-type hot sauce (limit to 1 teaspoon/day)
- Low-sodium baking powder
- Onion or garlic powder (avoid garlic salt)
- Tomato paste, unsalted tomatoes, unsalted tomato sauce
- Vinegar
- Water chestnuts
- Yeast
- Butter substitute (limit to ½ teaspoon/day)

Sweets

- Carob powder, cocoa powder
- Flavored gelatins
- Fruits
- Frozen juice bars, fruit ice, sorbet, sherbet
- Sugar, honey, molasses, syrup (cane or maple)
- Jelly, jam, preserves, apple butter
- Graham and animal crackers, fig bars, ginger snaps

Acknowledgments

I would like to thank my wife, Maria, and daughter, Eleanor, for their continued unwavering support.

Index

About the Author

Curtis Mark Rimmerman, MD, MBA, FACC is the initial holder of the Gus P. Karos Chair in Clinical Cardiovascular Medicine. He is a staff cardiologist and member of the Department of Cardiovascular Medicine and the Heart and Vascular Institute at the Cleveland Clinic, Cleveland, Ohio. He is certified by the American Board of Internal Medicine in Internal Medicine and the subspecialty of Cardiovascular Diseases. He is also certified by the National Board of Echocardiography and the American College of Physician Executives. His specialty interests include clinical cardiology, echocardiography, valvular heart disease, coronary artery disease, electrocardiography, and patient education.

Dr. Rimmerman, a native of Cleveland, Ohio, completed his undergraduate studies at Case Western Reserve University, graduating Magna Cum Laude with a degree in chemistry (Phi Beta Kappa). He spent his undergraduate junior year abroad through a scholarship at the University of Sussex in Brighton, England. He then returned to Case Western Reserve University where he graduated with the degree of Doctor of Medicine. Dr. Rimmerman completed his internship and residency in Internal Medicine at Vanderbilt University Medical Center in Nashville, Tennessee, followed by a Cardiology Fellowship at the Krannert Institute of Cardiology at Indiana University Medical Center in Indianapolis, Indiana. He continued his education while on staff at the Cleveland Clinic at the Case Western Reserve University Weatherhead School of Management, earning a Master's Degree in Business Administration.

Dr. Rimmerman was appointed to the Professional Staff of the Cleveland Clinic in 1993.

Nationally and internationally, Dr. Rimmerman has organized and chaired conferences and symposia on his specialty interests, with an emphasis on topics related to echocardiography. He has published articles and abstracts in leading medical journals on his specialty interests and authored or coauthored chapters in medical textbooks related to interactive electrocardiography, acute coronary syndromes, and myocardial infarction. His Interactive Electrocardiography CD-ROM and Workbook serves as an industry standard for electrocardiography education.

Dr. Rimmerman is a Fellow of the American College of Cardiology (FACC) and a member of the American Society of Echocardiography and certified member of the American College of Physician Executives.